Time to try....

the ULTIMATE BELLY BLITZ & BODY PLAN COOKBOOK

the essential body plan cookbook
delicious, quick & easy calorie controlled recipes plus ab
workout plan

Time to try... THE ULTIMATE BELLY BLITZ & BODY PLAN COOKBOOK

The essential body plan cookbook. Delicious, quick & easy calorie controlled recipes plus ab workout plan

ISBN 978-1-912511-93-8

DISCLAIMER

—— CONTENTS ——

Dinner Recipes

Snacks

Drinks

Ab Workouts & Stretches

INTRODUCTION

Regain that confidence in yourself, have fun cooking, planning and eating delicious, fresh and filling meals.

For many people, the main reason for refocusing on their diet and lifestyle with the aim of losing some weight is to achieve a flatter stomach. When we start making less healthy lifestyle and diet choices it quickly shows and there is no more obvious and immediate place for it to gather than our belly! This can be for many reasons, and whilst we all carry our weight, and excess weight differently, generally a larger belly is formed through our bodies' inability to properly digest processed or calorie-heavy foods. Many of these products are packed with artificial flavourings, calories, colourings or other chemicals and components that our digestive systems are just not used to, nor are they set up to cope with, and so our bodies turn it into fat and store it!

Therefore the best way to really effectively reduce that belly, get into better shape and also feel better in yourself is to go back to basics with fresh, natural, healthy and wholesome foods, focusing on a balanced diet with plenty of fruits and vegetables packed with nutrients and antioxidants.

A flat stomach cannot be achieved through diet alone; as much as our plates need to be balanced, so does our lifestyle and regular exercise is a key element of that. Many people are put off by the concept of 'regular exercise', demotivated and convinced that this must entail training for a marathon or competing at a high standard, yet this is not the case at all. An extensive variety of exercises can be undertaken, suited to you, to help you maintain a healthy and balanced life style. This does not need to be through an expensive gym membership, or an overly enthusiastic running club that clashes with meetings or dinner, but can quite simply be moderate workouts that can be easily followed in the privacy and security of your own home.

The core workouts provided in this book give a range of exercises that you can do each day to get your blood pumping, release those feel-good endorphins and specifically target the stomach area. They are handpicked and tailored exclusively with the aim of tightening up your core, burning tummy fat, and strengthening up those muscles to build up and improve your strength and fitness, regardless where you begin.

These core workouts, combined with a healthy and nutritious diet, are the absolute key to shifting an unwanted belly and keeping it off! Crash and fad diets do not work long term; they are unsustainable and many followers report that they end up with a larger tummy than they started with. When the crash diet ends, or you fall off track, your body often regains this lost weight in pure fat. The best way to approach weight loss and management is a healthy, natural and a balanced diet alongside exercises.

A huge part of this is monitoring portion control and calorie control. This brings a great level of awareness of what you are eating and how many calories are actually in the foods you are eating. When you begin paying attention you may be surprised; many foods that you may think are high in calories, are in fact not, and vice versa.

Eating a calorie deficit is the key to losing weight. This needn't be an aggressive calorie deficit. To begin with we would suggest 300 calories below your current intake. The recommended calorie intake to maintain your weight is approximately 2000 calories per day. So using a moderate deficit of 300 calories means you would consume no more than 1700 calories per day.

Our recipes give you a wealth of ideas to help plan your meals and show that monitoring your calorie intake is not as restrictive and unenjoyable as you would think. These recipes are full of vibrancy, colour, flavour and variety. Calorie controlled meals enable you to eat a huge range of foods – you are not required to completely eliminate anything, allowing you to enjoy your favourite foods through swapping some products for healthier versions, or simply refraining from overeating with inappropriate portion sizes.

Do you love your carbs and find nothing better than a warm bowl of pasta? Are you a real meat lover and couldn't bear to be deprived of a good rump steak every now and then or do you love a good dollop of mayo with your sweet potato wedges? Then this recipe book is for you as nothing is ultimately eradiated from your diet. It's just about making healthier choices and with so many meal plan ideas you could have dinner decided for months.

Allow yourself time to enjoy being back in the kitchen, making your own marinades and sauces to add flavour to your foods rather than off the shelf jarred sauces which are typically high in calories and salt. This does not need to be complicated either – it's really very simply! Many delicious foods, herbs, spices, fruits and vegetables can add instant flavour to a dish to leave your taste buds tingling for more. It needn't be time consuming either; many of these recipes can be prepared in advance and include a range of juices, drinks and smoothies to give you an energy boost whilst on-the-go.

Regain that confidence in yourself, have fun cooking, planning and eating delicious, fresh and filling meals. Be kind to your body and let yourself enjoy the exercises, even if it's just for 5 or 10 minutes a day, because that can make so much difference; little and often! And, even more importantly, enjoy seeing the results! This collection of recipes is designed to complement the core workouts, purposefully including ingredients that are rich in antioxidants and work brilliantly as anti-inflammatories, aiding digestion. The better your digestive system is working, the better you will feel, and the less bloated your stomach will be too.

Get yourself feeling fabulous again and there is no better time to start than today.

Time to try....

ULTIMATE BELLY BLITZ

BREAKFAST RECIPES

NOT-SO-NAUGHTY CHOCO & BANANA PORRIDGE

274 calories per serving

Ingredients

- 40g/1½oz organic porridge oats
- 250ml/8½fl oz unsweetened almond milk
- 1 small banana, peeled
- 1 tsp organic dark chocolate, grated

Method

1 Add the porridge oats and almond milk into a small saucepan and mix together on a low heat.

2 Gently stir the mixture continuously until it begins to thicken and the oats soften.

3 In a small bowl, mash half of the banana with a fork until a lumpy mixture is created. Cut the remaining half of the banana into thin slices and place to one side.

4 Add the mashed banana and half the grated dark chocolate into the pan of porridge and continue to gently stir through for 1 – 2 minutes.

5 Remove from the pan and serve. Arrange the sliced banana on top and sprinkle across the remaining dark chocolate.

CHEF'S NOTE

Almond milk is a brilliant, low-calorie alternative to cow's milk and still acts as a good source of calcium.

CHILLI TOMATOES ON TOAST

107
calories per serving

Ingredients

- 100g/3½oz tinned plum tomatoes, chopped
- A large pinch of chilli powder
- A pinch of fresh garlic, grated
- 1 tsp tomato puree

- 1 slice of wholegrain seeded bread
- A large pinch of chilli flakes
- ½ tsp linseeds
- A pinch of ground black pepper

Method

1 Place the chopped tomatoes in a bowl and mash gently with a fork or small masher until a chunky mixture is formed.

2 Add in the chilli powder, garlic and tomato puree and mix well.

3 Lightly toast or grill the bread and place on a plate to serve.

4 Spread the tomato mixture across the toast and top with a large pinch of chilli flakes. Sprinkle across the linseeds, season with black pepper and serve.

CHEF'S NOTE
This simple but nutritious breakfast is kept even lower in calories as no butter is needed – flavourful toast spreads and toppings are a great way to fill up but keep your stomach slim.

ENERGISING EGG AVOCADO

323

calories per
serving

Ingredients

- 1 small ripe avocado, halved and de-stoned
- 2 small eggs
- A dash of olive oil

- A small pinch of sea salt and pepper
- A large pinch of chilli flakes to serve
- A dash of freshly squeezed lime juice

Method

1 Pre-heat the oven to 180C/350F/Gas 4.

2 Place each half of the avocado in a roasting tray. Break one egg and carefully pour the yolk and white into the small hole where the avocado seed would have been embedded in one half. Repeat this method using the second egg for the other half.

3 Gently brush the avocado with a dash of olive oil and season with sea salt and pepper.

4 Place in the oven and cook for 15 minutes. Remove from the oven and top with chilli flakes and a squeeze of lime juice to serve.

CHEF'S NOTE

Prepare this super easy, energy-filled breakfast and allow to cook while you do your morning core work out.

SUPER CREAMY SCRAMBLED EGG ON TOAST

269 calories per serving

······· *Ingredients* ·······

- 2 small eggs
- 1 tbsp low-fat crème fraiche
- A small pinch of sea salt and pepper

- 1 tsp butter
- 1 slice of wholegrain, seeded bread

······· *Method* ·······

1 Crack the eggs into a bowl and beat together using a fork or small whisk.

2 Add in the low-fat crème fraiche and continue to whisk until the mixture is combined and well-aired. Season with salt and pepper and whisk once more.

3 Lightly toast or grill the bread.

4 Place a small saucepan on a medium heat and allow the butter to melt. Pour in the egg mixture. Whisk the mixture every 10 – 20 seconds to create a fluffy scrambled egg mixture and to prevent the mixture from burning or sticking to the bottom of the pan.

5 Cook until the mixture is no longer a liquid and spoon the scrambled egg mixture on top of the toast to serve.

CHEF'S NOTE

Eggs are an excellent source of protein and vitamin D that will help your body to grow stronger, complementing the core workouts wonderfully.

ZESTY LEMON AND HONEY GRANOLA YOGHURT

167
calories per serving

Ingredients

- ½ lemon
- 2 tbsp low-fat, natural yoghurt
- 1tsp honey
- 25g/1oz granola

Method

1 Lightly grate the zest of most of the lemon skin into a bowl, squeeze the juice into another and place to one side.

2 Spoon the yoghurt into a bowl and drizzle in around a quarter of the freshly squeezed lemon juice. Drizzle in the honey and stir the mixture together well.

3 Add in a small pinch of the lemon zest and stir once more.

4 Pour the lemon and honey yoghurt mixture over the granola and serve with an extra sprinkling of lemon zest on top to garnish.

CHEF'S NOTE

Lemon has many therapeutic qualities and is low in calories allowing you to add instant flavour to food with almost zero calorific impact.

PEANUT BUTTER AND BANANA WAFFLE

281 calories per serving

Ingredients

- 1 small banana, peeled and chopped
- 2 tsp low-fat peanut butter
- 1 fresh egg waffle
- 1 tsp flaxseeds

Method

1 Place the banana slices into a bowl and mash with a fork until a lumpy mixture is created.

2 Spoon in the peanut butter and mix well.

3 Lightly toast or grill the waffle to warm through and lightly crisp.

4 Spread across the banana and peanut butter mixture.

5 Sprinkle on top some flaxseeds to serve.

CHEF'S NOTE

Peanuts are a great source of unsaturated fats which, in moderation, can help lower cholesterol levels and improve general health.

SKINNY TOAST AND CHILLI MUSHROOMS

188 calories per serving

Ingredients

- 1 tsp extra virgin olive oil
- 100g/3½oz button mushrooms, finely chopped
- A pinch of chilli powder
- ¼ small red chilli, de-seeded and finely chopped
- 1 wholemeal pitta bread
- A pinch of fresh coriander, chopped

Method

1 Pre-heat the grill to a medium heat.

2 Place a frying pan on a medium heat with the olive oil. Add in the mushrooms and cook for 4 minutes, stirring occasionally.

3 Add in the chilli powder and chopped chilli, stir and allow to cook for further 2 – 3 minutes, or until the mushrooms and chilli have softened and are turning golden.

4 Meanwhile place the pitta bread under the grill to lightly toast.

5 Remove from the heat and cut open the pitta bread. Place each half on a plate to serve and top with the mushroom and chilli mixture from the pan.

6 Sprinkle on top the fresh coriander to serve.

CHEF'S NOTE

Chillies are thought to be a natural pain reliever and also an effective method of reducing blood cholesterol.

BERRY AND GRANOLA EXPLOSION

233
calories per serving

Ingredients

- 20g/¾oz blueberries
- 20g/¾oz raspberries
- 40g/1½oz oat granola (calories based on Kellogg's Original Granola)

- 1 tsp low fat natural Greek-style yoghurt
- ½ tsp honey
- A pinch of chia seeds

Method

1 Place the blueberries and strawberries into a bowl and gently mash with a fork until a lumpy, mush mixture is formed

2 Place the granola in a bowl and spoon on top the natural yoghurt.

3 Drizzle over the honey, stirring it into the yoghurt. Now, spoon on the prepared berry mixture and finish with a sprinkling of chia seeds to serve.

CHEF'S NOTE

Blueberries and raspberries are packed with antioxidants to help boost your immune system and bring a natural shine and strength to hair and nails.

TRADITIONAL HAM AND CHEESE OMELETTE

249
calories per serving

···· *Ingredients* ····

- 2 small eggs
- 1 tsp of whole milk
- A small pinch of dried nutmeg, ground
- A small pinch of sea salt and pepper

- 1 thin slice of lean ham
- 1 tbsp Parmesan, finely grated
- 1 tsp olive oil

···· *Method* ····

1 Crack the eggs into a bowl and beat them together with the milk using a fork or small whisk.

2 Add in the ground nutmeg, as well as the salt and pepper to season, and whisk well, adding air into the mixture.

3 Tear the slice of ham into small pieces and add into the mixture along with the grated Parmesan cheese and stir well. Bring a small pan to warm with the olive oil.

4 Once warmed through, pour in the egg mixture and cook for 2 – 3 minutes.

5 Carefully flip the omelette and cook on the other side for 1 – 2 minutes.

6 Remove from the heat and fold the omelette to serve.

CHEF'S NOTE

Omelettes are a brilliant, low-calorie way to kickstart your day with an energising, protein-based breakfast that is really quick and easy.

300 CALORIE ENGLISH BREAKFAST

300 calories per serving

Ingredients

- 1 lean pork chipolata sausage
- ½ medium tomato
- 1 tsp virgin olive oil
- 25g/1oz button mushrooms, chopped

- 1 rasher of lean bacon, fat removed
- 1 small egg
- 1 small slice of wholemeal bread
- 1 scrape of butter

Method

1 Pre-heat the grill to a medium heat. Place the sausage under the grill and cook for 5 minutes, or until the meat is beginning to golden and crisp slightly. Turn the sausage over and place back under the grill with the tomato half and bacon until cooked through.

2 Meanwhile, warm a small frying pan on a medium heat with the oil. Add in the chopped mushrooms and cook for 3 - 5 minutes, stirring occasionally.

3 Move the mushrooms to the side of the pan, crack in the egg and cook for 2 – 3 minutes, or until the egg white is cooked through. Flip the egg and cook to your liking.

4 Toast the slice of bread and add a very light spread of butter. Place on a plate and serve with the cooked breakfast.

CHEF'S NOTE

An English breakfast can provide a good, balanced boost to your diet and does not need to be high in calories; you can even reduce this to less than 200 calories by losing the buttered toast!

THE GREEN BIG ENGLISH

300
calories per
serving

···· Ingredients ····

- 25g/1oz kale
- ½ medium tomato
- 2 rashers of lean bacon, fat removed
- 1 tsp olive oil

- 2 small eggs
- ½ small avocado, peeled, de-stoned and sliced

···· Method ····

1 Pre-warm the grill to a medium heat and bring a pan of water to boil. Place a steamer on top of the pan and add in the kale. Steam for 7 – 10 minutes, until the kale is cooked through and tender.

2 Meanwhile, place the tomato under the grill and cook for 3 minutes. Add the rashers of bacon under the grill and cook for a further 2 – 3 minutes.

3 While the bacon and tomatoes cook, warm a small frying pan on a medium heat and add the oil. Crack the eggs into the pan and allow to cook for 3 – 5 minutes, while you turn the bacon over, rotate the tomato and allow them to cook for another 2 – 3 minutes.

4 Once the egg whites have cooked through, either remove from the pan to serve, or, if you prefer a

less runny yolk, cook for a further 2 – 3 minutes, or flip the egg and cook for 1 – 2 minutes.

5 Remove the kale from the steamer, or drain if boiled, and serve with the bacon, tomato and eggs. Place alongside the breakfast the prepared avocado and serve.

CHEF'S NOTE
Avocadoes are high in potassium and really aid digestion to reduce inflammation; combine this with a core workout and you will see remarkable results for your tummy.

QUICK & EASY
KICKSTARTER HAM & EGG

182
calories per
serving

Ingredients

- 2 small eggs
- ½ tbsp semi-skimmed milk
- A small pinch of sea salt and pepper
- Dash of olive oil

- 1 slice of thick cut lean ham
- A small pinch of fresh chives, finely chopped

Method

1 Pre-warm a small frying pan to a medium heat with the oil.

2 In a small jug, crack the eggs and whisk well. Pour in the milk, season with salt and pepper and whisk once more.

3 Pour the egg mixture into the pan, gently stir the mixture with a spatula and allow to cook for 30 seconds. Stir the mixture again to prevent it from settling or sticking to the bottom of the pan. Repeat this until a fluffy, scrambled egg mixture is created.

4 Place the slice of ham on a plate and serve alongside the warm scrambled egg. Add a sprinkling of chives on top to serve.

CHEF'S NOTE

This super simple breakfast is so quick to prepare and gives you a protein-fuelled kickstart to the day. Add a pinch of chilli powder to the scrambled egg for a spicy twist!

SMOKED SALMON ON-THE-GO HOTBOX

254
calories per serving

Ingredients

- 2 small eggs
- Dash of olive oil
- ½ tbsp semi-skimmed milk
- A small pinch of sea salt and pepper
- 40g/1½oz fresh smoked salmon

- A splash of freshly squeezed lemon juice
- ½ small avocado, peeled, de-stoned and sliced
- A small pinch of fresh chives, finely chopped

Method

1 Place to one side a small Tupperware pot.

2 Pre-warm a small frying pan to a medium heat with the oil.

3 In a small jug, crack the eggs and whisk well. Pour in the milk, season with salt and pepper, whisk once more and add to the pan.

4 Gently stir the mixture with a spatula and allow to cook for 30 seconds. Stir the mixture again to prevent it from settling or sticking to the bottom of the pan. Repeat this until a fluffy, scrambled egg mixture is created.

5 Place the smoked salmon in the Tupperware pot with a quick squeeze of fresh lemon juice.

6 Layer on top the sliced avocado. Then, spoon the scrambled egg from the pan on top of the avocado and sprinkle on the chopped chives.

7 Eat as you go or place the lid on top and enjoy as soon as you can.

CHEF'S NOTE

It's not always easy to find time to cook and eat breakfast; this quick-to-cook on the go option allows you time to squeeze in a core work out, and still get your body a nutrient-filled breakfast.

SUPER LOW-CALORIE GREEN OMELETTE

189 calories per serving

Ingredients

- 2 small eggs
- 1 tsp of whole milk
- A small pinch of sea salt and pepper
- 1 tsp low-fat green pesto
- 25g/1oz spinach
- Dash of virgin olive oil

Method

1 Crack the eggs into a bowl, using both the egg and yolk and beat them together with the milk using a fork or small whisk.

2 Add in the salt and pepper to season and whisk well adding air into the mixture. Add in the green pesto and whisk well once more until the pesto is smoothly combined with the egg mixture.

3 Tear the spinach leaves into smaller pieces and add into the egg and pesto omelette mixture and stir well.

4 Put a small pan on a medium heat with the oil.

5 Once warmed through, pour in the egg mixture and cook for 2 – 3 minutes, or until golden brown underneath and the top of the mixture is mainly cooked with little runny mixture left.

6 Carefully turn the omelette and cook on the other side for 1 – 2 minutes. Remove from the heat and fold the omelette to serve.

CHEF'S NOTE

Spinach is a really effective way of giving your diet a quick and easy injection of iron, boosting your energy levels, and can be used in so many different ways.

MANGO AND POMEGRANATE PORRIDGE

205 calories per serving

Ingredients

- 40g/1½oz organic porridge oats
- 250ml/8½fl oz unsweetened almond milk
- 25g/1oz fresh mango, peeled and chopped
- 20g/¾oz fresh pomegranate, peeled and chopped
- A pinch of dried, ground cinnamon

Method

1 Add the porridge oats and almond milk into a small saucepan and mix together on a low heat.

2 Gently stir the mixture continuously until it begins to thicken and the oats soften.

3 You can either add the fresh, chopped fruit into the porridge in the pan, stirring continuously to warm through, or simply serve the porridge in a bowl and top with the fresh fruit for a nice, cool contrast. Sprinkle on top a pinch of cinnamon to serve.

CHEF'S NOTE

Porridge is high in fibre that is excellent for digestion, helping to reduce inflammation and bloating and allowing you to see the results from the core workouts quicker.

SUPER LOW-CALORIE RED BERRY YOGHURT

52
calories per serving

Ingredients

- 2 fresh strawberries, finely chopped
- 5 fresh raspberries, finely chopped
- 25g/1oz fresh cranberries

- 60g/2½oz low-fat, natural yoghurt
- 1 fresh mint leaf, finely chopped

Method

1 Place the strawberries, raspberries and cranberries in a bowl and mash together with a fork until a lumpy, juicy coulis-style texture is created.

2 Spoon in the yoghurt and mix well to combine with the red berry mixture.

3 Sprinkle on top the freshly chopped mint and simply serve as it is, or place in a small container to eat on-the-go if need be.

CHEF'S NOTE

This can easily be prepared the night before and stored in the fridge to allow you more time for your morning core workout.

ROASTED MUSHROOM STUFFED TOMATOES

143 calories per serving

Ingredients

- 7g/¼oz butter
- ½ small clove of garlic, minced
- 100g/3½oz button mushrooms, finely chopped

- ½ tbsp crème fraiche
- 1 large tomato, halved
- Dash of olive oil

Method

1 Pre-heat the oven to 180C/350F/Gas 4.

2 In a frying pan melt the butter on a medium heat. Add in the garlic and mushrooms and cook for 5 - 7 minutes, until the mushrooms begin to soften.

3 Remove the mixture from the pan and place in a food processor, or in a bowl if using a hand blender. Give the mixture a few blasts to create a relatively smooth mixture, but not completely pureed.

4 Spoon in the crème fraiche to the mushroom mixture and stir well by hand.

5 Delicately scoop out the inside of the tomato halves and spoon in the creamy mushroom mixture.

6 Lightly brush with olive oil and place on a baking tray. Cook in the oven for 10 – 15 minutes, or until the tomato skins soften and the tops begin to crisp.

CHEF'S NOTE

Mushrooms are a powerful antioxidant, boosting your immune system, and are incredibly low in calories and fat.

VIBRANT FRUIT GRANOLA

322 calories per serving

Ingredients

- 50g/2oz granola
- 1 kiwi, de-skinned and chopped
- 20g/¾oz blueberries
- 20g/¾oz raspberries
- 100g/3½oz low-fat Greek-style yoghurt

Method

1 Pour the granola into a bowl.

2 Toss together the chopped kiwi and berries and place on top of the granola.

3 Spoon on top either Greek yoghurt, or a Greek-style, low-fat yoghurt and serve.

4 For a juicy alternative, mash together the fruit and stir into the yoghurt before serving with the granola.

CHEF'S NOTE

Kiwi adds a great tropical flavour to simple dishes and aids digestion that, along with core workout exercises, can deliver excellent results for achieving a flatter tummy.

FRUIT AND NUTTY YOGHURT

204
calories per serving

Ingredients

- 100g/3½oz low-fat, natural yoghurt
- 5 almonds, chopped or crushed
- 5 hazelnuts, chopped or crushed
- 15g/½oz raisins
- 1 tsp honey

Method

1 Spoon the yoghurt into a bowl ready to serve.

2 Sprinkle in the majority of the chopped/crushed nuts, leaving some to sprinkle on top.

3 Stir well and then add in the raisins, stirring the mixture one more.

4 Drizzle over the honey to sweeten the yoghurt and top with the leftover crushed nuts to serve.

CHEF'S NOTE
Whilst typically high in calories, when eaten in small portions, nuts contain a wealth of nutrients to improve blood pressure levels and general heart health.

TROPICAL FRUIT SALAD

122
calories per
serving

Ingredients

- 50g/2oz watermelon, skin removed & diced
- 50g/2oz pineapple, skin removed & diced
- 1 kiwi, skin removed, sliced & halved
- 1 clementine, peeled
- 3 strawberries, stalk removed & quartered
- 1 tsp honey

Method

1 Place the prepared fruit into a bowl and gently toss together, mixing the fruit around to create a gorgeously colourful fruit salad.

2 In a small separate bowl, mash the strawberries with a fork until a smooth texture is formed.

3 Pour in the honey and mix well with the strawberries to create a sweet but fruity sauce to add to the fruit salad.

4 Drizzle the sweet strawberry juice over the fruit salad and serve.

CHEF'S NOTE

Many tropical fruits are less sugary and acidic than some traditional British fruits; their high water content can bring a new vibrancy to your skin.

WATER MELON SALAD

277 calories per serving

Ingredients

- 50g/2oz low fat Feta cheese, crumbled
- 250g/9oz watermelon flesh, cubed
- 50g/2oz fresh peas
- 75g/3oz baby courgettes/zucchini

- 1 tbsp lemon juice
- 1 tsp olive oil
- 1 tbsp chopped fresh mint
- ½ tsp crushed chilli flakes

Method

1 Preheat the grill to medium/high.

2 Slice the baby courgettes lengthways and place on the grill, flesh side up.

3 Season both well, sprinkle with chilli flakes and spray with a little low cal cooking spray.

4 Grill for 2-3 minutes each side or until golden.

5 In a bowl mix together the mint, olive oil, cubed watermelon, fresh peas (eat these raw) and lemon juice.

6 Arrange on a plate with the crumbled cheese and courgettes/zucchini.

CHEF'S NOTE
Low fat Feta cheese is a great diet ingredient; full of flavour and goodness.

Time to try....

ULTIMATE BELLY BLITZ

LUNCH RECIPES

AVOCADO PRAWN MESS

317
calories per serving

Ingredients

- 1 tbsp low-fat mayonnaise
- 1 tsp tomato ketchup
- 1 tsp salad cream
- 75g/3oz fresh prawns, cooked and de-shelled

- 1 small avocado, skin removed, halved and de-stoned
- 1 large pinch of fresh chives, finely chopped
- 1 large lemon wedge

Method

1 Add the low-fat mayonnaise, ketchup and salad cream into a bowl and mix well until a pink, Marie Rose-style sauce is created.

2 Add in the prawns and stir them into the sauce well.

3 Place the avocado halves on a plate ready to serve. Spoon the prawn mixture into the holes where the avocado stone would have sat, and then spoon the remaining mixture on top, allowing it to spill out over the avocado.

4 Garnish with freshly chopped chives and serve with a fresh, chunky wedge of lemon.

CHEF'S NOTE

Avocado has many health benefits, one of which is to reduce bloating, aiding the appearance of a flatter tummy.

CURRIED WINTER CARROT SOUP

133 calories per serving

Ingredients

- 1 tsp olive oil
- 60g/2½oz onion, peeled and finely chopped
- 300g/11oz carrots, peeled and chopped
- 500ml/2 cups vegetable stock
- 2 tsp mild curry powder
- A pinch of ground nutmeg
- A large pinch of salt and pepper
- 1 tsp natural yoghurt
- A pinch of fresh coriander, finely chopped

Method

1 Place the oil into a saucepan and warm on a medium heat.

2 Add in the onion and carrots and cook for 2 – 3 minutes until the onion and carrot edges are beginning to soften.

3 Add in the stock, stir well and simmer for 2 – 3 minutes.

4 Add in the curry powder and nutmeg, season with salt and pepper, give a final stir and then reduce the heat to simmer for 35 – 40 minutes.

5 Either pour the soup into a food processor or use a hand blender to blitz the soup into a smooth, lump-free consistency ready to serve. Pour into a bowl and drizzle on top some of the natural yoghurt, followed by a sprinkling of fresh coriander to serve.

CHEF'S NOTE

Curry powder has a wealth of nutritional benefits and is renowned for relieving inflammation.

ONION SOUP

237
calories per
serving

···· *Ingredients* ····

- 30g/1oz butter
- 450g/1lb onions, peeled and finely sliced
- 1 clove of garlic, minced
- 300ml/10½fl oz vegetable stock

- 100ml/3½fl oz dry white wine
- A splash of freshly squeezed lemon juice
- A large pinch of salt and pepper
- A pinch of sugar

···· *Method* ····

1 Place a saucepan on a medium heat and add in the butter.

2 Once the butter has half melted add in the chopped onion and stir it into the butter so it is evenly coated.

3 Allow the onions to simmer for 1 – 2 minutes, stirring occasionally. Next, add in the garlic and simmer for a further 1 – 2 minutes. Pour in the vegetable stock, stirring well to prevent the onion from clumping together at the bottom and simmer for 4 – 5 minutes.

4 Pour in the white wine along with the splash of lemon juice and season well with salt and pepper. Add a sprinkling of sugar and stir one final time before reducing the heat slightly so the soup is simmering, not bubbling, and leave it to simmer for 25 – 30 minutes. Remove from the heat and serve.

CHEF'S NOTE

Onions are packed with phytochemicals that are good for your immune system, keeping your body as strong as possible.

RED LENTIL AND CHILLI SOUP

308 calories per serving

Ingredients

- 1 tsp olive oil
- 40g/1½oz onion, finely chopped
- ½ clove of garlic, minced
- 25g/1oz celery, finely chopped
- 25g/1oz carrots, peeled and chopped
- 400ml/14fl oz vegetable stock
- 150g/5oz red lentils
- 1 small red chilli, de-seeded and finely chopped
- 60ml/2fl oz red wine
- A pinch of chilli flakes

Method

1 Place a saucepan on a medium heat with the oil.

2 Add in the chopped onion and garlic and simmer for 1 – 2 minutes, stirring regularly to prevent them from sticking to the pan.

3 Add in the chopped celery and carrot and simmer again for 1 – 2 minutes, stirring regularly so that the sliced vegetables are turned over to brown on each side, where possible.

4 Pour in the vegetable stock and stir well so that the vegetables do not all sit at the bottom. Next, add in the red lentils and chilli, stir well, and allow the soup to simmer for 4 – 5 minutes.

5 Pour in the red wine, stir once more, and reduce the heat so that the soup is simmering only, not bubbling, and leave for 25 – 30 minutes.

6 Remove from the heat, pour into a bowl and sprinkle some chilli flakes on top to serve.

CHEF'S NOTE

Red Lentils are a brilliant source of fibre that help regulate bowel movements, consequently reducing bloating or inflammation from constipation, helping your tummy to look and feel slimmer.

LEEK, POTATO AND BACON SOUP

268 calories per serving

Ingredients

- 1 tsp virgin olive oil
- 2 rashers of bacon, fat removed and finely chopped
- 60g/2½oz onion, peeled and finely sliced
- 150g/5oz leeks, sliced

- 500ml/17½fl oz vegetable stock
- 400g/14oz potatoes, peeled and chopped
- 1 tsp dried mixed herbs
- A large pinch of pepper
- 100ml/3½fl semi-skimmed milk

Method

1 Place a saucepan on a medium heat with the oil.

2 Allow the oil to warm and add in the bacon. Cook for 1 – 2 minutes and then add in the chopped onion and leeks.

3 Cook the vegetables for 2 – 3 minutes, so they soften slightly, stirring regularly. Pour in the vegetable stock and bring to a boil.

4 Add the chopped potatoes and mixed herbs, season well with pepper and then reduce the heat slightly to a simmer, rather than a boil, and simmer for 35 – 40 minutes, stirring occasionally.

5 Pour in the milk and stir well, allowing it to warm through.

6 Pour into a food processor to blend to a smooth texture. Serve immediately.

CHEF'S NOTE

Leeks have many health benefits and are rich in Vitamin K which helps your body to regulate bloody flow – this is important during core work outs to enable you to get the most from your core exercises.

MUSHROOM AND SWEETCORN SOUP

185 calories per serving

Ingredients

- 15g/½oz butter
- 50g/2oz onion, peeled and finely chopped
- 75g/3oz button mushrooms, finely sliced
- 200ml/7fl oz vegetable stock
- 150g/5oz tinned sweetcorn
- 100ml/3½fl oz semi-skimmed milk
- A large pinch of sea salt and pepper
- ½ tbsp low-fat crème fraiche

Method

1 Place a saucepan on a medium heat and add in the butter. Once the butter is half melted add in the onion and mushrooms, stirring well, and cook for 2 – 3 minutes.

2 Once starting to soften, pour in the vegetable stock and bring to a simmer, altering the heat to ensure the soup is only simmering, now boiling.

3 Mix in the sweetcorn and allow the soup to simmer for 30 – 35 minutes. Using a hand blender or food processor, blend the mixture until a smooth consistency as possible, and then return to the pan.

4 Pour in the milk and season well with salt and pepper. Stir well and allow to simmer for another 3 – 4 minutes. Serve straight from the pan and enjoy whilst warm and drizzle on top some crème fraiche to serve.

CHEF'S NOTE

Mushrooms have a wealth of nutritional and health benefits and can help to aid weight loss when combined with exercises in your core workouts.

HALLOUMI AND MANGO SALAD

342 calories per serving

·········· *Ingredients* ··········

- 1 tsp extra virgin olive oil
- A large splash of freshly squeezed lime juice
- A large splash of freshly squeezed lemon juice
- A pinch of salt and pepper
- 50g/2oz halloumi, sliced

- 75g/3oz baby leaf salad
- 50g/2oz ripe mango, skin removed, de-stoned and chopped
- 25g/1oz ripe avocado, peeled, de-seeded and chopped
- 7g/¼oz pine nuts

·········· *Method* ··········

1 Pour the olive oil into a small bowl and mix with the lime and lemon juice.

2 Season with salt and pepper, stir once more and place to one side to use as the salad dressing.

3 Place a small frying pan on a medium heat and add in the halloumi slices. Make sure you do not add any oil or butter to the pan as Halloumi cooks best dry.

4 Cook for 2 – 3 minutes, or until the halloumi begins to 'sweat' on top. Turn the halloumi over and repeat on the other side. Continue to turn and cook for 30 seconds to 1 minute until the halloumi begins to golden.

5 Toss the salad leaves, mango and avocado in a bowl ready to serve.

6 Place the cooked halloumi on top and drizzle over the dressing.

7 Top with a sprinkling of pine nuts to serve.

CHEF'S NOTE

Mango is fantastic for your skin, leaving you glowing even more after those core workouts.

CLASSICALLY SIMPLE WALDORF SALAD

210 calories per serving

Ingredients

- 1 tbsp low-fat soured cream
- ½ tsp honey
- A small pinch of salt and pepper
- ½ green apple, cored and sliced
- ½ celery stick, finely chopped
- 100g/3½oz lettuce leaves, chopped
- 15g/½oz raisins
- 15g/½oz walnuts, de-shelled and crushed

Method

1 Spoon the sour cream into a bowl and drizzle in the honey.

2 Season with salt and pepper, mix together and place to one side to use as the salad dressing shortly. Toss in a bowl together the apple, celery and lettuce.

3 Add in the prepared salary dressing and toss the salad again so it is evenly covered.

4 Sprinkle in the raisins and walnuts and toss one final time before serving.

CHEF'S NOTE

Apple makes a great addition to salad and has good prebiotic effects, aiding digestion and helping your tummy to stay flatter.

SUPER SIMPLE LOW-CAL GREEK SALAD

177 calories per serving

Ingredients

- 75g/3oz cucumber, sliced and halved
- 75g/3oz red onion, peeled and chopped
- 75g/3oz cherry tomatoes, halved
- 75g/3oz mixed pitted olives, halved
- A large splash of freshly squeezed lemon juice
- A large pinch of pepper
- 75g/3oz feta cheese, cubed

Method

1 Place the chopped cucumber, red onion and tomatoes in a bowl and toss well together.

2 Add in the chopped olives and mix once more, allowing the natural oils from the olives to spread around the salad.

3 Add in a good splash of freshly squeezed lemon juice and a good pinch of pepper and mix well once more.

4 Top with the cubed feta cheese, allowing it to crumble slightly as it is thrown into the salad. Using your hands, gently mix the salad together and serve.

CHEF'S NOTE

This super simple salad is quick and easy to prepare, is packed with natural oils and antioxidants and is great to use any leftovers for a side salad at dinner.

BACON AND AVOCADO WARM SALAD

245 calories per serving

Ingredients

- 2 rashers of lean bacon, fat removed
- ½ tsp extra virgin olive oil
- A large splash of freshly squeezed lemon juice
- A pinch of salt and pepper

- 50g/2oz lettuce leaves, chopped
- 50g/2oz avocado, peeled, de-stoned and chopped
- 50g/2oz cherry tomatoes, chopped

Method

1 Pre-heat the grill to a medium heat. Place the rashers of bacon with the fat removed on a grill tray that allows the fat to drop down when cooking, rather than the bacon sitting in its own fat, and place under the grill for 2 – 3 minutes.

2 Turn the bacon over and return to the grill for a further 2 – 3 minutes, or until cooked through.

3 Mix the olive oil, lemon juice and salt and pepper in a small bowl and place to one side to use as a simple salad dressing.

4 Place the chopped lettuce, avocado and tomatoes in a bowl and toss well.

5 Chop the cooked bacon up, either into strips or square pieces, depending on your preference, and add to the tossed salad.

6 Drizzle as little or as much of the prepared dressing as you like and serve whilst warm.

CHEF'S NOTE

Bacon adds instant flavour to any salad and dramatically decreases in calories when the fat is removed and it is grilled, rather than fried.

RAW ENDIVE, WHITE ONION AND LEMON SALAD

82 calories per serving

······· *Ingredients* ·······

- ½ tsp extra virgin olive oil
- ½ tsp freshly squeezed lemon juice
- ½ tsp honey
- ½ tsp water
- A pinch of sea salt and pepper

- A pinch of lemon zest, grated
- 100g/3½oz endive, chopped
- 75g/3oz onion, peeled and finely chopped
- 25g/1oz alfalfa sprouts

······· *Method* ·······

1 Pour the olive oil and lemon juice into a small bowl and gently mix together to form the base of the salad dressing.

2 Drizzle in the honey and next add the water, mixing well.

3 Sprinkle in the sea salt and pepper, along with the freshly grated lemon zest and stir the dressing well. Place to one side ready to use shortly – it is more than likely that you will not require all of the dressing.

4 Place the chopped endive into a bowl along with the chopped onion and alfalfa sprouts and toss well. Drizzle in roughly a quarter of the prepared dressing and toss well.

5 Add in a little more dressing and mix once more to serve.

CHEF'S NOTE

Endive is brilliantly low in calories and can really aid digestion to help keep you feeling energised for those core workouts and achieve the flat belly you have always dreamed of.

CARROT, TOMATO AND GINGER SOUP

67 calories per serving

Ingredients

- 1 tsp olive oil
- ½ small red onion, peeled and finely chopped
- 2 large carrots, peeled and chopped
- A pinch of fresh root ginger, grated

- 200g/7oz tinned chopped tomatoes
- 175ml/6fl oz vegetable stock
- 1 small bay leaf
- A pinch of dried mixed herbs
- A pinch of salt and pepper

Method

1 Place a saucepan on a medium heat with the oil.

2 Add in the chopped onion and stir around the pan so the pieces are covered in the oil and simmer for 1 minute.

3 Add in the chopped carrot and ginger and simmer for another 1 - 2 minutes, stirring every now and then.

4 Pour in the tinned tomatoes and a quarter of the vegetable stock, mix well and simmer for 2 to 3 minutes.

5 Pour in the remaining vegetable stock, stirring well, and then add in the bay leaf, mixed herbs and season with salt and pepper.

6 Reduce the heat slightly and allow the soup to simmer, not boil, for 35 – 40 minutes.

7 Either serve the soup as it is for a chunky soup texture, or remove the bay leaf and use a hand blender or food processor to reduce to a smooth, lump-free texture if preferred.

CHEF'S NOTE

Carrots are great for your immune and digestive systems.

TOMATO AND HAM RED OMELETTE

189 calories per serving

Ingredients

- 2 small eggs
- 1 tsp of whole milk
- A small pinch of sea salt and pepper
- 1 tbsp passata

- 3 cherry tomatoes, quartered
- 1 thin slice of lean ham
- 1 tbsp low-fat cheddar cheese
- 1 tap olive oil

Method

1 Crack the eggs into a bowl and beat them together with the milk using a fork or small whisk. Add in the salt and pepper to season and whisk well adding air into the mixture.

2 Spoon in the passata and mix well; this is what will give the omelette its red colour.

3 Add in the chopped tomatoes and tear the slice of ham into small pieces before also adding into the mixture. Sprinkle in the grated cheese and mix gently.

4 Put a small pan on a medium heat with the oil. Once warmed through, pour in the egg mixture and cook for 2 – 3 minutes, or until golden brown underneath and the top of the mixture is mainly cooked with little runny mixture left.

5 Carefully turn the omelette and cook on the other side for 1 – 2 minutes. Remove from the heat and fold the omelette to serve.

CHEF'S NOTE

Tomatoes are not only very low in calories, but they are also high in antioxidants, helping your body to ward off illnesses and disease, staying stronger for longer and aiding weight loss.

SMOKED SALMON RYEBREAD

213 calories per serving

Ingredients

- 40g/1½oz cucumber, shredded
- 40g/1½oz low-fat cream cheese
- A large splash of freshly squeezed lemon juice
- A pinch of black pepper
- 2 slices of ryebread
- 50g/2oz fresh smoked salmon
- A large pinch of fresh chives, finely chopped
- 1 small wedge of lemon

Method

1 Spoon the shredded cucumber into a bowl and gently fold into the cream cheese.

2 Stir in the freshly squeezed lemon juice as well as the pepper.

3 Spread the cream cheese mixture thickly onto the ryebread slices.

4 Twist, fold or tear the salmon to arrange on top of the creamed ryebread.

5 Garnish with freshly chopped chives and serve with a small wedge of lemon to add extra juice if required.

CHEF'S NOTE

Adding lemon can instantly add flavour or a twist to almost any marinade, dressing or salad and is an effective means of aiding indigestion and encouraging weight loss.

SWEET POTATO JACKET AND CHILLI TUNA MAYO

274 calories per serving

Ingredients

- 1 large sweet potato
- 1 spray of extra virgin olive oil
- A pinch of sea salt
- 50g/2oz tinned tuna

- ½ tbsp low-fat mayonnaise
- A pinch of salt and pepper
- A pinch of chilli powder
- A pinch of chilli flakes

Method

1 Pre-heat the oven to 200C/400F/Gas 6.

2 Pierce the potato several times with a knife all over and spray with the oil.

3 Using your hands rub the oil all over the potato and season with salt.

4 Place the potato on a baking tray and cook for 40 - 45 minutes, rotating the potato half way through, or until the sweet potato is crisp on the outside, but light and fluffy on the inside.

5 Meanwhile, spoon the tuna into a bowl along with the mayonnaise, salt and pepper and chilli powder.

6 Mix the ingredients well together to create a light tuna mayonnaise. Place to one side ready to serve.

7 Remove from the baked potato from oven and slice open.

8 Spoon in the tuna mayonnaise mixture and sprinkle on top the chilli flakes to serve.

CHEF'S NOTE

This is a perfect, warm and filling lunch for cold, winter days to maintain your energy levels, boosting your workouts, without overloading on calories.

Time to try....

ULTIMATE BELLY BLITZ

DINNER RECIPES

CREAMY SPINACH STUFFED MUSHROOMS

110 calories per serving

Ingredients

- 75g/ 3oz onion, peeled and finely chopped
- 400g/14oz spinach
- 1 tbsp low-fat crème fraiche

- A pinch of fresh parsley, finely chopped
- A pinch of ground black pepper
- 4 large flat mushrooms
- 1 tbsp parmesan cheese, grated

Method

1 Pre-heat the oven to 180C/350F/Gas 4.

2 Bring a pan of water to boil to steam, or boil if preferred, the vegetables. Add in the onion and allow to cook for 2 – 3 minutes before adding in the spinach.

3 Steam or boil for 3 – 5 minutes, or until the spinach is softened and wilting and the onions softened.

4 Drain and place the spinach and onion in a bowl.

5 Add in the crème fraiche, parsley and pepper to season and mix well.

6 Place the mushrooms facing up on a baking tray and scoop out any remaining stalk. Spoon in the creamy spinach mixture.

7 Place in the oven for 10 – 15 minutes. Remove from the oven and sprinkle on top the grated parmesan cheese.

8 Return to the oven and cook for a further 5 – 10 minutes, until the cheese is beginning to crisp. Remove from the oven and serve.

CHEF'S NOTE

Ingredients such as spinach and mushroom really aid digestion and help to reduce bloating.

CHICKEN TIKKA PARCELS

270

calories per serving

Ingredients

- ½ tsp root ginger, grated
- ½ clove of garlic, minced
- 1 tsp fresh coriander, finely chopped
- ½ tsp chilli powder
- A pinch of ground turmeric
- A pinch of salt

- 1 tbsp freshly squeezed lemon juice
- 75g/3oz low-fat natural yoghurt
- 1 tsp honey
- 200g/7oz chicken fillets, diced
- 100g/3½oz brown rice
- ½ little gem lettuce, leaves separated

Method

1 Place the ginger, garlic, coriander, spices and salt in a bowl and toss together. Add in the lemon juice, yoghurt and honey and stir well to make a tikka marinade for the chicken.

2 Add the diced chicken into the marinade. Ideally, cover and allow the chicken to rest in the marinade for as long as possible; making in this in the morning and allowing to marinade throughout the day in the fridge achieves the best flavour.

3 Pre-heat the oven to 170C/325F/Gas 3. Place the marinated chicken into an oven dish and pour on top all of the remaining marinade. Cover with a lid of tin foil and cook for 30 – 40 minutes, until the chicken is tender and cooked through.

4 Meanwhile, bring a pan of water to boil and add the rice. Simmer for 15 – 20 minutes, or until tender.

5 Arrange several of the little gem lettuce leaves on a plate, ready to serve.

6 Drain the rice and spoon into each leaf a small portion of rice as a base for the tikka parcel. Remove the chicken tikka from the oven and spoon the chicken on top of the rice, ready to serve.

CHEF'S NOTE

Many spices contain strong antioxidants and have anti-inflammatory properties reducing the appearance of bloating.

PEANUT BUTTER NOODLES

379
calories per serving

Ingredients

- 75g/3oz cherry tomatoes, finely chopped
- 40g/1½oz tbsp smooth peanut butter
- 1 tbsp tomato puree
- A large pinch of chilli flakes
- A large pinch of chilli powder
- 200g/7oz free egg noodles
- 3 tbsp low-fat crème fraiche
- 15g/½oz plain peanuts, crushed

Method

1 Place a small saucepan on a medium heat and add in the cherry tomatoes. Add in the smooth peanut butter and stir well to combine it with the tomatoes.

2 Spoon in the tomato puree and then add in the chilli flakes and powder, stirring well again and allowing the mixture to simmer for 1 – 2 minutes.

3 Add in the egg noodles and fold the sauce over them so they are evenly covered and allow them to cook for 3 – 4 minutes, or the advised time if otherwise stated on the packaging.

4 Stir continuously to avoid them sticking to the bottom of the pan, adding in the peanuts, and eventually the crème fraiche.

5 Warm the sauce through and serve straight from the pan.

CHEF'S NOTE
Noodles are typically a complex carbohydrate, an ideal way to keep you feeling full and energised for busy afternoons.

SUPER SIMPLE LEMON AND HERB STUFFED CHICKEN

313 calories per serving

Ingredients

- ½ tbsp low-fat cream cheese
- ½ clove of garlic, minced
- ½ tsp mixed herbs
- A pinch of salt and pepper
- 1 free-range medium chicken breast

- 1 fresh lemon wedge
- 100g/3½oz Maris Piper potatoes, peeled and chopped
- 1 tbsp low-fat crème fraiche

Method

1 Pre-heat the oven to 180C/350F/Gas 4. In a small bowl spoon in the cream cheese. Add in the minced garlic and mixed herbs, season with salt and pepper, and stir well.

2 Slice the chicken breast down its side, as if you were intending to cut it in half, but not completely doing so; cut the breast deep enough that you can spread the mixture but that the breast does not half or split and separate.

3 On top of the spread, place the lemon wedge, inside the breast, and close the breast back up. Place on a square of tin foil, big enough so that you can fold the edges to cover the chicken into a small parcel to steam cook in the oven. Once completely wrapped, place the chicken in the oven and cook for 35 – 40 minutes.

4 Meanwhile, bring a saucepan of water to boil and add in the chopped potatoes. Boil on a medium heat for 25 – 30 minutes, or until the potatoes are cooked through and tender. Remove from the heat and drain.

5 Return the potatoes to the pan and mash them well. Spoon in the crème fraiche, mixing well, and cover to keep warm until serving.

6 Once cooked, peel back the tin foil from the chicken carefully; open slightly at first to allow the steam to escape. Place on a plate and serve along with the mashed potato. Use any juices collected in the tinfoil to drizzle on top and serve.

HONEY MUSTARD SAUSAGES & SWEET POTATO MASH

190 calories per serving

·········· Ingredients ··········

- 2 low-fat pork sausages
- ½ tbsp honey
- ½ tbsp wholegrain mustard

- 100g/3½oz sweet potatoes, peeled and chopped
- A splash of freshly squeezed lemon juice

·········· Method ··········

1 Pre-heat the oven to 350F (gas mark 4). Place the sausages in a small roasting dish and smother in the honey and whole grain mustard, using a spoon to combine the two ingredients and evenly cover the sausages. Pierce the sausages once or twice each and then place in the oven for 10 – 15 minutes.

2 Meanwhile, bring a pan of water to boil and add in the sweet potato. Boil for 25 minutes, or until the potatoes are cooked through. Turn the sausages over to ensure they cook evenly and do not burn on top and spoon the honey and mustard around the roasting dish again to cover the sausages. Return the sausages to the oven for a further 15 – 20 minutes, or until cooked through and starting to crisp. Once cooked, drain the sweet potatoes and return them to the pan to mash.

3 Add in a dash of freshly squeezed lemon juice, mash, and then cover to keep warm until the sausages are thoroughly cooked.

4 Spoon the sweet potato mash onto a plate and serve with the sausages arranged on top. Drizzle over any remaining honey and mustard sauce from the roasting dish and serve.

CHEF'S NOTE

Sweet potatoes are a good source of fibre and are a great alternative to normal potatoes.

ROASTED BEETROOT AND WARM ORANGE SALAD

123 calories per serving

Ingredients

- 1 medium beetroot
- 1 spray of olive oil
- A pinch of sea salt and pepper
- 40g/1½oz fresh rocket leaves
- ½ orange, peeled and segments separated
- 20g/¾oz red onion, peeled and finely chopped
- 25g/1oz feta cheese, cut into small cubes

Method

1 Pre-heat the oven to 180C/350F/Gas 4.

2 Place the beetroot on a roasting tin and spray with the oil. Sprinkle on a pinch of salt and pepper to season and rub all over the beetroot so it is evenly oiled and seasoned. Roast in the oven for 30 – 35 minutes.

3 Remove from the oven and allow to cool for 5 minutes. Then, peel off the beetroot skin and chop into cubes.

4 Toss in a bowl together the rocket leaves, orange segments, red onion and feta cubes. Add in the chopped roasted beetroot and toss once more before serving.

CHEF'S NOTE

Beetroot adds immediate colour and flavour to any meal and is excellent for improving digestion and relieving constipation; both of which can make your stomach bloat if left untreated.

TUNA STEAK AND PEPPER SALAD

279 calories per serving

Ingredients

- 25g/1oz red pepper, stalk removed, de-seeded and finely diced
- 25g/1oz yellow pepper, stalk removed, de-seeded and finely diced
- 25g/1oz red onion, peeled and finely diced
- 25g/1oz cherry tomatoes, finely chopped

- A pinch of fresh coriander, finely chopped
- 1 tsp extra virgin olive oil
- A splash of freshly squeezed lime juice
- 1 tsp olive oil
- 125g/4oz fresh tuna steak
- 40g/1½oz fresh rocket leaves

Method

1 Place the chopped red pepper, yellow pepper, red onion and tomatoes in a small bowl and mix well to begin making a simple salsa style salad. Add in the finely chopped coriander along with the olive oil and splash of fresh lime juice. Stir well and place to one side ready to serve shortly.

2 Place a small frying pan on a high heat with the oil.

3 Add the tuna steak to the pan. Allow to cook for 2 minutes and then flip over and cook on the other side for a further 2 minutes or until the tuna steak is cooked to your preference.

4 Place the rocket leaves on a plate to serve and spoon the chopped pepper salsa style mixture into the middle to act as a bed for the tuna steak.

5 Remove the cooked tuna steak from the pan and serve immediately, placing on top of the pepper salsa salad and enjoy.

CHEF'S NOTE

Tuna is rich in a variety of vitamins and minerals, namely Omega-3, and is excellent for your heart.

ROASTED ASPARAGUS AND WALNUT SALAD

243 calories per serving

Ingredients

- 100g/3½oz asparagus stalks, chopped
- 2 sprays olive oil
- A large pinch of salt and pepper to season
- 50g/2oz fresh baby leaf salad
- 25g/1oz cherry tomatoes, chopped
- 15g/½oz walnuts, shelled and chopped
- 25g/1oz avocado, peeled, de-stoned and diced
- 1 tsp extra virgin olive oil
- A splash of freshly squeezed lemon juice

Method

1 Pre-heat the oven to 180C/350F/Gas 4.

2 Place the asparagus stalks in a roasting dish and spray with the oil. Season well with sea salt and pepper and mix the asparagus around the dish so it is evenly covered in oil and seasoning.

3 Roast in the oven for 20 – 25 minutes, or until cooked through and the ends are beginning to crisp slightly.

4 In a bowl add the baby leaf salad, chopped tomatoes and avocado.

5 Toss well together and add in the walnuts.

6 Pour in the olive oil and a splash of fresh lemon juice and mix the salad together well once more.

7 Once cooked, remove the asparagus from the oven, add into the salad, mix well and serve whilst warm for maximum flavour.

CHEF'S NOTE

Asparagus is brilliant for reducing bloating and adding more folate to your diet.

GRILLED CHICKEN AND CREAMY BEAN RICE

366 calories per serving

Ingredients

- 50g/2oz long grain brown rice
- 40g/1½oz green beans, chopped
- 125g/4oz chicken breast
- 40g/1½oz frozen green peas

- 1 tbsp low-fat crème fraiche
- 25ml/1fl oz white wine
- A large pinch of salt and pepper

Method

1 Pre-heat the grill to a medium heat. Bring a pan of water to boil.

2 Add in the brown rice and simmer for 3 – 4 minutes. Add in the chopped green beans and simmer for 5 minutes.

3 Meanwhile, place the chicken breast on a tray and grill for 4 – 5 minutes. Add the frozen peas to the saucepan and continue to simmer for a further 10 minutes. Remove from the grill, turn the breast over and cook for a further 10 minutes or until cooked through.

4 Continue to cook the rice and beans until the rice is thoroughly cooked through and the beans and peas are tender.

5 Remove from the heat and drain well. Return the rice, beans and peas to the saucepan, but not the heat just yet, and spoon in the crème fraiche. Pour in the white wine and season with salt and pepper.

6 Mix the crème fraiche, wine and seasoning into the rice mixture, stirring well, and return to a low heat to warm through; stir continuously to prevent the mixture from burning or sticking to the bottom of the pan.

7 Once warmed through, remove from the heat and spoon onto a plate ready to serve. Place the grilled chicken on top of the rice and bean mixture and serve.

ORANGE, SESAME & GINGER BEEF & SPRING ONION RICE

346 calories per serving

Ingredients

- 1 tsp freshly squeezed orange juice
- ½ tsp fresh orange zest, grated
- A splash of light soy sauce
- ½ tsp fresh root ginger, grated
- ½ clove of garlic, minced

- 100g/3½ oz long grain rice
- 1 100g lean rump steak, fat removed
- 2 spring onions, finely sliced
- 1 tsp sesame seeds

Method

1 Squeeze the orange juice into a bowl and add in the orange zest and soy sauce. Mix together well and add in the grated ginger and garlic. Place a small pan on a medium heat and add in the orange and ginger mixture. Allow it to warm through and simmer for 1 – 2 minutes.

2 Remove from the heat and spoon the mixture, and all juices, onto the rump steak. Using the back of a spoon, cover the rump steak in the mixture, turning over to cover both sides.

3 Bring a pan of water to boil and add in the long grain rice. Boil until tender stirring occasionally to prevent the rice from sticking to the bottom of the pan.

4 Meanwhile, place a frying pan on a medium heat and add in the marinated rump steak, along with any marinade that may have drained off in the transfer to the pan. Cook for 2 – 3 minutes, or until the steak begins to 'sweat' on top. Turn the steak over and repeat on the other side. Continue to cook to your preference. Once cooked, boil the kettle and remove the rice from the heat. Drain the rice and pour the boiled water over the rice to get rid of any excess starch.

5 Return the rice to the pan and add in the finely sliced spring onion. Spoon the rice then onto a plate ready to serve. Place the cooked rump from the pan on top of the rice and drizzle over the remaining juices from the pan, sprinkle on top the sesame seeds and serve immediately.

SIMPLE MARGHERITA PITTA PIZZA WITH WEDGES

435 calories per serving

Ingredients

- 100g/3½oz sweet potato, peeled and cut into wedges
- 2 sprays olive oil
- A pinch of sea salt
- 1 wholemeal pitta bread

- 2 tbsp passata
- 40g/1½oz low-fat cheddar cheese, grated
- 2 cherry tomatoes, sliced
- A large pinch of pepper

Method

1 Pre-heat the oven to 180C/350F/Gas 4.

2 Place the sweet potato wedges on a roasting tray and squirt with the oil. Turn the wedges over, rolling them in the oil to ensure an as even coverage as possible and season with sea salt. Cook in the oven for 25 – 30 minutes. Meanwhile, prepare the pitta pizzas.

3 Either place the pitta bread under the grill for 1 - 2 minutes on each side or use a toaster to cook it until it opens inside and is almost crisping on the outside.

4 Slice the pitta into half, cutting it open sideways so you have to full size halves, rather than cutting the pitta into semi-circle halves, opening it out and being careful to allow the steam to escape first.

5 This will act as your pizza base. Spoon onto each of the pitta slices the passata and spread around the slices so there is even coverage but stopping roughly half a centimetre from the edges. Sprinkle on top the cheese and top with the tomato halves.

6 Season with pepper and place in the oven for 5 – 10 minutes, or until the cheese has melted and the edges are beginning to crisp. Remove the sweet potato wedges and pitta pizza from oven and serve immediately whilst warm.

ROASTED BUTTERNUT SQUASH RISOTTO

183 calories per serving

Ingredients

- 150g/5oz butternut squash, peeled and diced
- 50g/2oz carrot, peeled and chopped
- 1 tsp extra virgin olive oil
- 1 litre/1½ pints water
- 150g /5oz quinoa, rinsed
- ½ tsp ground nutmeg
- 1½ tbsp low-fat crème fraiche
- A splash of freshly squeezed lemon juice
- A pinch of salt and pepper

Method

1 Pre-heat the oven to 180C/350F/Gas 4.

2 Toss the butternut squash and carrot in the olive oil and place in a roasting dish. Roast for 30 – 35 minutes, stirring the vegetables half way through, turning over pieces where necessary.

3 Meanwhile, prepare the quinoa. Bring the water to boil in a saucepan. Add in the quinoa and a pinch of salt simmer for 10 minutes, stirring continuously.

4 Sprinkle in the nutmeg and allow the quinoa to simmer for a further 5 minutes, or until fully cooked and expanded.

5 When cooked, drain any excess water and mix in the crème fraiche and splash of lemon juice. Season with salt and pepper and add in the roasted butternut squash and carrot.

6 Mix well and return to the heat to warm through. Best served straight from the pan.

CHEF'S NOTE

Quinoa makes a brilliant risotto alternative to traditional rice and contains an almost endless list of nutritious benefits with its exceptionally high protein, fibre and mineral content.

SMOKEY BACON AND TOMATO PASTA

246
calories per serving

Ingredients

- 125g/4oz wholemeal pasta
- 1 tsp olive oil
- 2 rashers of smoked bacon, fat removed, chopped
- 200g/7oz tinned tomatoes
- 1 tbsp tomato puree
- 1 tsp chilli powder
- 1 tsp ground paprika
- 2 tbsp low-fat crème fraiche
- A pinch of fresh coriander, finely chopped

Method

1 Bring a pan of water to boil and add in the fusilli pasta. Boil for 10 – 12 minutes, or until the pasta is thoroughly cooked. Meanwhile add the oil to a frying pan and add in the chopped smoked bacon. Cook for 2 – 3 minutes, or until the pieces are cooked through, stirring to ensure they do not burn or stick to the pan.

2 Add in the tinned tomatoes, stir, and allow to simmer for 2 minutes. Spoon in the tomato puree and mix well.

3 Allow to simmer for a further 2 minutes. Add in the spices, again, mixing well, and reduce the heat to a low temperature and leave the mixture to summer for 3 – 4 minutes, only stirring when it begins to bubble a little.

4 Once cooked, drain the pasta and then place it back in the saucepan. Pour the tomato and bacon mixture from the frying pan into the saucepan and fold the pasta into the sauce gently, before giving a good stir.

5 Return the pan to a low heat and add in the crème fraiche. Mix well, warm through and serve with a fresh coriander garnish.

CHEF'S NOTE

Spices such as chilli and paprika are good for your metabolism and can really aid digestion and inflammation, helping to keep your tummy feeling smoother and looking thinner.

GARLIC HERB CHICKEN AND BUTTERED PEAS

297
calories per serving

Ingredients

- 1 tsp extra virgin olive oil
- 1 clove of garlic, minced
- A large pinch of dried mixed herbs
- 125g/4oz chicken breast

- 75g/3oz green beans, chopped
- 75g/3oz frozen peas
- 7g/¼oz butter
- A large pinch of salt and pepper

Method

1 Pre-heat the oven to 180C/350F/Gas 4.

2 In a small bowl pour in the olive oil. Add in the minced garlic and mixed herbs and stir well. Place the chicken breast on a piece of tin foil large enough to cover and wrap up the breast.

3 Smother the chicken breast in the garlic and herb oil marinade and wrap the tin foil so the chicken breast is completely covered. If you have time, place the breast to one side or in the fridge to marinade for as long as possible to achieve a richer flavour.

4 Place in the oven and cook for 35 – 40 minutes. Meanwhile, bring a pan of water to boil. Add in the chopped green beans and boil for 10 minutes.

5 Add in the peas and boil for a further 10 minutes. Once cooked through and tender, drain the beans and peas and place in a small roasting tin.

6 Spoon in the butter, allowing it to melt over the greens, and stir well so the greens are fairly evenly covered in the melted butter. Season well with salt and pepper and place in the oven for the final 5 minutes of the chicken breast cooking.

7 Remove all from the oven. Unwrap the chicken, being careful to allow the steam to first escape, and place onto a plate ready to serve. Spoon over as much of the juices and excess marinade from the tin foil as possible. Then, spoon the buttered beans and peas onto the plate and serve immediately.

TOMATO AND GOATS CHEESE FILO TARTS

128
calories per serving

Ingredients

- 1 sheet of Jus-Rol filo pastry
- 1 egg white
- 1 medium tomato, sliced
- A large pinch of dried basil

- 40g/1½ oz low-fat goats cheese
- A pinch of salt and pepper
- 1 tbsp low-fat cheddar cheese, grated
- Fresh basil leaves to garnish

Method

1 Allow the pastry to sit at room temperature to soften for 1 – 2 hours prior to preparing and cooking.Pre-heat the oven to 200C/400F/Gas 6). Roll out the pastry and cut the sheet into quarters. Lightly brush the pastry with egg white and discard any remaining egg white unused.

2 Place one of the pastry quarters into a muffin tin and layer with a second quarter. Repeat this for the remaining two quarters.

3 Place one fine slice of tomato in each tartlet base and add a little of the basil. Spoon on top some of the goats cheese and season with salt and pepper. Add on top another slice of tomato, a sprinkling of basil, and some more goats cheese. Repeat once more for each tartlet.

4 Sprinkle on top the cheddar cheese, along with some torn basil leaves. Place in the oven and cook for 12 – 15 minutes, or until the pastry has risen and is crisp, and the tomatoes softened through. Serve with a fresh rocket salad.

CHEF'S NOTE

Goats cheese is often easier to digest than normal cheese, reducing bloating and keeping your tummy looking slim.

Time to try....

ULTIMATE BELLY BLITZ

SNACK RECIPES

WHOLEMEAL PITTA STRIPS AND HUMMUS

222
calories per serving

Ingredients

- 150g/5oz tinned chickpeas, drained
- ½ clove of garlic, crushed
- 2 tsp tahini paste
- 25ml/1fl oz vegetable stock
- 2 tsp olive oil
- 1 tbsp freshly squeezed lemon juice
- A pinch of salt and pepper
- 2 small wholemeal pitta breads
- 1 tsp Branston pickle

Method

1 Place the drained chickpeas in a food processor.

2 Add in the garlic and tahini paste and blend well together.

3 Add in half of the vegetable stock and the olive oil and blend again.

4 Next, add in the remaining stock and oil, along with the lemon juice, season with salt and pepper and blend again until a smooth, thick mixture is created.

5 Spoon into a bowl and place to one side ready to serve.

6 Toast or grill the pitta breads until lightly crisped.

7 Chop the pittas into strips and serve next to the hummus. Spoon the Branston pickle on top of the hummus and enjoy.

CHEF'S NOTE

Chickpeas are an excellent source of fibre, helping to regulate blood sugar levels and improve the strength of your heart.

SWEET POTATO WEDGES & ROASTED GARLIC MAYO

172 calories per serving

Ingredients

- 200g/7oz sweet potato, peeled and chopped
- 2 sprays of extra virgin olive oil
- A pinch of sea salt

- 2 cloves of garlic
- 3 tbsp low-fat mayonnaise
- A splash of freshly squeezed lemon juice
- A pinch of fresh coriander, finely chopped

Method

1 Pre-heat the oven to 180C/350F/Gas 4.

2 Place the sweet potato wedges on a roasting tray and spray with the oil.

3 Turn the wedges over, rolling them in the oil to ensure an as even coverage as possible and season with sea salt.

4 Wrap the 2 garlic cloves in tin foil and place on the baking tray as well. Remove the garlic from the over after 20 minutes but allow the sweet potatoes to roast for a further 15 – 20 minutes.

5 Meanwhile, prepare the mayonnaise dip; allow the garlic cloves to cool slightly and then squeeze out the caramelised garlic into a bowl.

6 Spoon in the low-fat mayonnaise and stir well. Add in the lemon juice and fresh coriander, mix well and place in a small bowl ready to serve.

7 Once cooked and beginning to crisp, remove the sweet potato wedges from the oven and serve with the garlic mayo dip.

CHEF'S NOTE

Sweet potatoes are good for the heart and this is a brilliant snack or side to fill you up and give you an energy boost for any mid-morning or afternoon core workouts.

CHEESE AND RED ONION STRAWS

185 calories per serving

·········· *Ingredients* ··········

- 60ml/2floz warm water
- A large pinch of dried yeast
- 1 tsp olive oil
- ½ red onion, finely chopped
- 100g/3½oz strong white flour

- A pinch of salt
- A small pinch of dried sage
- A small pinch of dried rosemary
- 1 tbsp Parmesan cheese, grated

·········· *Method* ··········

1 Pre-heat the oven to 220C/425F/Gas 7. Keep the warm water in a jug and sprinkle in the dried yeast. Whisk the yeast into the water and rest.

2 Meanwhile place the oil into a small frying pan and cook the red onion for 5 minutes on a medium heat, or until softened.

3 Sieve the flour into a bowl and mix in the salt and herbs. Add in most of the Parmesan cheese. Mix the ingredients together, adding in the red onion.

4 Next, pour in a third of the yeast and water mixture and stir well. Gradually add in the remaining water and yeast mixture. Knead the mixture to create a dough. Add a splash of water or sprinkling of flour as needed to achieve a good dough consistency.

5 Remove the dough from the bowl and place on a surface dusted with a little flour and knead well for 3 – 5 minutes, Place the dough back into the bowl, cover with a damp tea towel or cloth and leave to breathe and rise for 1 – 2 hours. If you can, leave a little longer.

6 Return the dough to the floured surface and knead once more. Then, roll the dough out so that it is roughly 1cm thick and cut into sticks; the length and width of which to your preference. Roll up any edges unused into another dough ball and repeat the process to utilise all of the dough.

7 Place each 'stick' of dough onto a baking tray and lightly slice the top of each one and top with the remaining parmesan cheese. Bake in the oven for 20 – 25 minutes, or until risen, golden and crisp.

LEMON ROASTED ASPARAGUS & PARMA HAM

119 calories per serving

Ingredients

- ¼ lemon
- ½ tsp sunflower oil
- A pinch of salt and pepper

- 8 stalks of asparagus
- 3 slices of Parma ham
- ½ tsp linseeds

Method

1 Pre-heat the oven to 200C/400F/Gas 6.

2 Give the lemon a good squeeze and collect the juice in a bowl. Add in the salt and pepper, mix well and place to one side. Either brush the oil and lemon juice mixture over each stalk, or lightly roll them in the oil, and place on a baking tray.

3 Cook in the oven for 20 – 25 minutes or until the asparagus is tender. Cool for a few minutes before serving.

4 Tear the Parma ham up into small pieces and sprinkle on top of the asparagus to serve with a sprinkling of linseeds to garnish.

CHEF'S NOTE

Asparagus helps to flush excess fluid and salt from the body, which complements core workouts in keeping your tummy looking trim.

PRAWN AND CUCUMBER BITES

67 calories per serving

Ingredients

- 100g/3½oz fresh prawns, cooked and shelled
- 40g/1½oz low-fat cream cheese
- ½ tsp freshly squeezed lemon juice
- ½ cucumber
- ½ tsp fresh chives, finely chopped

Method

1 Finely chop the prawns, or if preferred, give them a quick burst with a hand blender, to mince them down slightly to create a lump spread.

2 Mix with the low-fat cream cheese and lemon juice, stirring well.

3 Slice the cucumber and use as a base to create bite-sized snacks.

4 Spoon some of the creamy prawn mixture on top of each slice of cucumber and garnish with freshly chopped chives to serve.

CHEF'S NOTE

Prawns have an enormous range of health benefits, the most notable being their high selenium content which has been linked to the prevention of some cancers.

STUFFED CELERY STICKS

93 calories per serving

················· *Ingredients* ·················

- 100g/3½oz low-fat cottage cheese
- 1 tsp freshly squeezed lemon juice
- ½ clove of garlic, minced
- 1 tsp fresh chives, finely chopped

- 15g/½oz walnuts, crushed
- 4 celery sticks
- A pinch of chilli powder

················· *Method* ·················

1 Spoon the cottage cheese into a small bowl and pour in the freshly squeezed lemon juice.

2 Stir well before adding in the garlic, chives and the majority of the walnuts – leave a large pinch aside to sprinkle on top later.

3 Mix the ingredients together. Spoon the mixture onto each celery stick, spreading it along the stick to fill the ridge.

4 Sprinkle the leftover crushed walnuts on top of the cottage cheese stuffing and light dust with chilli powder to serve.

CHEF'S NOTE

Celery contains antioxidants that can reduce inflammation.

ROOT VEGETABLE CRISPS

87
calories per
serving

················ *Ingredients* ················

- 1 tsp extra virgin olive oil
- 150g/5oz sweet potatoes, peeled and finely sliced
- 150g/5oz beetroot, peeled and finely sliced
- 150g/5oz carrots, peeled and finely sliced
- 100g/3½oz parsnips, peeled and finely sliced
- A large pinch of sea salt

················ *Method* ················

1 Pre-heat the oven to 200C/400F/Gas 6.

2 Lightly brush a baking tray with some of the olive oil. Place the vegetable slices on the baking tray, arranging them to fit as many on as possible. You may need several trays depending on the size of your oven and trays or need to reuse the same tray and run a few batches.

3 Lightly brush the slices with some more of the olive oil and season with salt. Cook for 15 to 20 minutes, or until the vegetables are nice and crisp.

4 Check the crisps halfway through cooking and shuffle them about to prevent them from sticking or turn some slices over if need be.

5 Serve straight away or store any unrequired portions in an air tight container.

CHEF'S NOTE

This is a brilliant natural alternative to typical high calorie crisps to satisfy that 'snacky' craving but help to keep your tummy flat.

MEDITERRANEAN OLIVES

113
calories per
serving

Ingredients

- ½ clove of garlic, minced
- ½ tsp freshly squeezed lemon juice
- ½ tsp extra virgin olive oil
- ½ tsp red wine vinegar
- 200g/7oz pitted olives
- 50g/2oz sundried tomatoes

- 25g/1oz red onion, peeled and finely chopped
- 7g/¼oz tsp pine nuts
- A pinch of fresh mint, finely chopped
- A pinch of fresh coriander, finely chopped
- A large pinch of salt and pepper

Method

1 Place the garlic, lemon juice, olive oil and red wine vinegar into a bowl and mix together well.

2 Add in the olives, stirring well, and then the sundried tomatoes and chopped onion.

3 Toss well so they are evenly covered in the lemon and garlicky oil marinade.

4 Next, sprinkle in the pine nuts along with the fresh herbs and salt and pepper to season.

5 Give the mixture one final stir and serve.

CHEF'S NOTE
Olives can effectively help to sustain and improve blood pressure levels.

SERRANO HAM AND WILD ROCKET

97 calories per serving

Ingredients

- 40g/1½oz fresh wild rocket leaves
- ½ tsp freshly squeezed orange juice
- A drizzle of extra virgin olive oil
- A pinch of salt and pepper
- 6 slices of Serrano ham

Method

1 Place the fresh rocket leaves in a bowl.

2 Pour in the freshly squeezed orange juice, along with the olive oil and salt and pepper.

3 Toss the salad well so the oil and orange juice are mixed over fairly evenly.

4 Spoon the rocket leaves onto a plate and use as a base for serving the Serrano ham. Twist or fold the ham on top of the rocket as you please to serve and enjoy.

CHEF'S NOTE

Serrano ham is highly nutritious and a good source of iron, making it an excellent energy boosting snack in between meetings or before a core workout.

APPLE, GRAPE AND RASPBERRY FRUIT POT

67 calories per serving

···················· *Ingredients* ····················

- ½ Pink Lady apple, cored and chopped
- 10 green grapes, halved
- 8 raspberries
- 1 tsp low-fat natural yoghurt
- A pinch of chia seeds

···················· *Method* ····················

1 Place the chopped apple, grapes and raspberries into a bowl, or if preparing to eat on-the-go or for later, place in a small pot or container.

2 Gently toss the chopped fruit together so it is evenly mixed up. Spoon on top the natural yoghurt, allowing it to drizzle down through the mixed fruit.

3 Top with a pinch of chia seeds and either enjoy or cover with a lid securely.

CHEF'S NOTE
Fruit makes a great, energising snack and can be easily prepared ahead and eaten on-the-go.

RICE CAKE WITH HOT CHILLI AVOCADO SMASH

216
calories per serving

······· *Ingredients* ·······

- ½ small avocado, peeled, de-seeded and mashed
- ½ tsp freshly squeezed lime juice
- 15g/½oz red onion, peeled and finely chopped

- A large pinch of salt and pepper
- A large pinch of tsp chilli powder
- ½ small red chilli, finely sliced
- 1 wholegrain low-fat rice cake
- A pinch of chilli flakes

······· *Method* ·······

1 In a bowl add the smashed avocado and lime juice and mix them together well.

2 Add in the onion, season with salt and pepper, and mix together.

3 Sprinkle in the chilli powder, along with the sliced red chilli, and stir well once more.

4 Spread the chilli avocado mixture onto the rice cake and top with chilli flakes to serve.

CHEF'S NOTE
Chilli is thought to be a great mood booster, putting you in the right frame of mind for your core workout routine.

Time to try....

ULTIMATE BELLY BLITZ

DRINKS RECIPES

STRAWBERRY AND LIME SMOOTHIE

86 calories per serving

Ingredients

- 100g/3½oz strawberries, de-stalked and chopped
- ½ small banana, peeled and chopped
- 1 lime
- 150ml/5floz almond milk

Method

1 Place the strawberries and banana in a bowl and mash together with a masher or large pestle and mortar.

2 Squeeze in the juice of 1 fresh lime and mix together. Add the fruit mixture into a food processor and blend together for 1 minute. Allow the mixture to rest and blend for a further 30 seconds.

3 Pour in half of the almond milk and blend again, before then repeating this process with the remaining almond milk until a smooth, combined mixture is created.

4 Either store in the fridge or serve straight away.

CHEF'S NOTE
Almond milk is a brilliant alternative to whole milk and can heavily aid digestion, reducing inflammation.

MANGO AND RASPBERRY SMOOTHIE

67
calories per serving

Ingredients

- 75g/3oz mango, peeled, de-seeded and chopped
- 25g/1oz raspberries
- 150ml/5fl oz semi-skimmed milk
- A splash of freshly squeezed lemon juice
- A small pinch of flaxseeds
- A pinch of pomegranate seeds

Method

1 Place the mango in a bowl and bash with the edge of a rolling pin, or use a small mallet if you have one, to soften the mango and mash slightly.

2 Add in the raspberries and give one last mashing. Add the fruit lumps, mush and all juices into a food processor and blend for 1 minute.

3 Pour in the milk and blend for a further 1 – 2 minutes. Next, add in the lemon juice, flaxseeds and pomegranate seeds and blend for a final 1 – 2 minutes.

4 Chill in the fridge and enjoy later or serve straight away.

CHEF'S NOTE

Mango is low in calories and helps to keep you hydrated.

KIWI BLAST

73
calories per
serving

······ *Ingredients* ······

- ¼ fresh lime
- 150g/5oz fresh kiwi, peeled and chopped
- 100g/3½oz cucumber, chopped
- 1 small banana, chopped
- 50ml/2fl oz water

······ *Method* ······

1 Squeeze the juice of a quarter of a lime into a small bowl and place to one side, ready to add to the drink shortly.

2 Place the chopped kiwi and cucumber into a food processor and blend for 1 minute or until a smooth juice is created.

3 Add in the chopped banana and half of the water and repeat for a further minute.

4 Pour in the remaining water and the fresh lime juice and blend one final time.

5 Serve straight away, or chill in the fridge to enjoy cold later on.

CHEF'S NOTE

Kiwi boosts your immune system and is brilliant for digestion, helping your body to stay strong and healthy and your stomach appear less bloated.

RICH BERRY BLITZ

57
calories per
serving

·············· *Ingredients* ··············

- ¼ fresh lime
- 50g/2oz raspberries
- 50g/2oz blueberries
- 50g/2oz blackberries

- 50g/2oz cranberries
- 1 small banana, chopped
- 150ml/5fl oz water
- 7g/¼oz tsp pomegranate seeds

·············· *Method* ··············

1 Squeeze the juice of a quarter of a lime into a small bowl and place to one side, ready to add to the drink shortly.

2 Place all of the berries into a bowl and gently mash together with a fork or a food masher.

3 Pour them into a food processor, including as much of the juices as possible.

4 Add in the chopped banana and blend for 1 – 2 minutes.

5 Give the mixture a good shake. Pour in the water and pomegranate seeds and blend for another 1 – 2 minutes.

6 Pour into a glass and enjoy right away, or chill to drink later.

CHEF'S NOTE

Berries are powerful antioxidants and can dramatically improve the appearance of skin, as well as strengthening hair and nails.

ZINGY CARROT AND GINGER JUICE

127
calories per serving

Ingredients

- 500g/1lb 2oz carrots, peeled and chopped
- 1 large orange, peeled and segments separated
- 50ml/2fl oz water
- 1 tsp fresh root ginger, grated
- 1 tsp honey
- ½ tsp flaxseeds

Method

1 Place the chopped carrots in a large pan of water and bring it to boil.

2 Boil for 20 – 25 minutes, or until the carrots are cooked and tender.

3 Drain the carrots and place them into a food processor ready to blend. Add in the orange segments, water and fresh ginger and blend for 1 – 2 minutes.

4 Allow the mixture to rest and blend again. Repeat until a smooth, lump-free mixture is created.

5 Next, drizzle in the honey and add in the flaxseeds. Give the mixture one last blend and serve.

CHEF'S NOTE

Carrots are believed to be a great anti-ageing food and can improve the appearance of skin; combine this with the core workouts and you will be left both feeling and looking great.

CITRUS TEA

10
calories per
serving

······ *Ingredients* ······

- 1 wedge of fresh lemon
- ½ tsp of freshly squeezed lemon juice
- ½ tsp of freshly squeezed orange juice

- 300ml/10½fl oz boiled water
- A splash of clear honey

······ *Method* ······

1 Gently pierce the lemon wedge and give it a soft squeeze so it begins to release some juice and can better infuse the tea.

2 Place the lemon wedge in a mug, along with the lemon juice and orange juice. Bring a kettle or pan of water to boil.

3 A typical mug will hold between 300 – 350ml of water, however this measurement does not need to be exact nor specifically measured – just use however much your mug will comfortably take for a cup of tea. Pour the water into your mug and gently stir so the lemon and orange juice mixes well with the water and the lemon wedge.

4 Add in the honey and stir gently for 30 seconds to 1 minute, or until the honey has melted into the water. The honey should take the edge off the bitterness of the citrus. Leave for 2 or 3 minutes to cool slightly before drinking.

CHEF'S NOTE

Lemon in hot water is renowned for kick-starting your metabolism and helping with weight loss; a great way to start your day with a citrus tea before a core workout.

SWEET AND SPARKLING GRAPEFRUIT JUICE

68 calories per serving

········· *Ingredients* ·········

- ½ grapefruit, peeled
- ½ pink lady apple, peeled, cored & chopped
- 3 strawberries, stems removed & chopped
- ½ tsp freshly squeezed lemon juice
- 150ml/5fl oz sparkling water

········· *Method* ·········

1 Separate the grapefruit segments or chop the fruit up into smaller pieces to place in a food processor.

2 Add in the apples and strawberries and blend for 30 seconds.

3 Add in the lemon juice and a large splash of the sparkling water. Blend for 1 – 2 minutes or until the fruits are smoothly blended together.

4 Pour in the remaining sparkling water and give the mixture a good mix. Blend the mixture one last time for 5 – 10 seconds to ensure thoroughly blended and serve.

CHEF'S NOTE

Grapefruit can kick-start your metabolism, however it can be quite bitter; the apple and strawberries act as a natural sweetener for this juice bursting with flavour.

Core WORKOUTS

Toning and building muscle in your core takes work and yes it can be tough. For the first few day you will likely suffer from tight and tender muscles in your abdominals but as you regularly exercise, this will ease and you will be able to focus on getting the best from your workouts.

We have compiled **3** core workouts to perform throughout each week. Choose one workout to perform per day and use the remaining 4 days to rest. Try to alternate between training and rest days. Each workout lasts for approximately 15 mins and a simple explanation of how to correctly perform each exercise in the set is explained in the following pages.

It is very important to warm up your muscles and joints before beginning any exercise to prevent injury and to make sure you perform each repetition to the best of your ability. Warm up by jogging on the spot for two minutes. Stand upright, with your feet shoulder-width apart. Contract and release your abdominal muscles for 15 to 20 repetitions to warm up your abs.

Always cool down and stretch at the end of your workout. Gently jog for 2 minutes then stretch out your core by performing the cobra and cat & cow stretches. (see page 96).

Tips

- Warm up and cool down before and after each workout
- Have a bottle of water to drink from between sets
- Remember to breathe through each exercise
- Keep your core tight

Core WORKOUT ONE

- Exercise 1: **BICYCLE CRUNCH** 30 secs | 10 secs rest
- Exercise 2: **LEG RAISE** 30 secs | 10 secs rest
- Exercise 3: **STANDING SIDE CRUNCH** 30 secs | 10 secs rest
- Exercise 4: **T STABILASTION** 30 secs | 10 secs rest
- Exercise 5: **JUMPING JACK** Hold position for 15 secs then reverse position for a further 15 secs | 10 secs rest
- Exercise 6: **V – UP** 30 secs | 2 minute rest

Repeat for 2 more sets

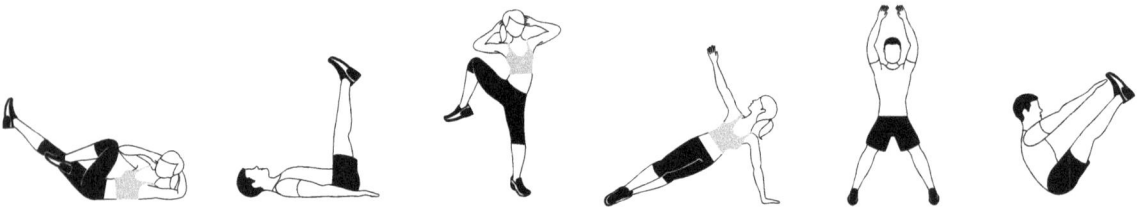

Perform each exercise as many times as possible within 30 seconds or hold for the desired length of time depending on the drill. Rest for 10 seconds then perform the next exercise again for 30 secs with a 10 sec rest in between exercises. Repeat until all 6 exercises have been completed.

Rest for 2 minutes then repeat the whole set two more times with a 2 minute rest in between.

Bicycle CRUNCH

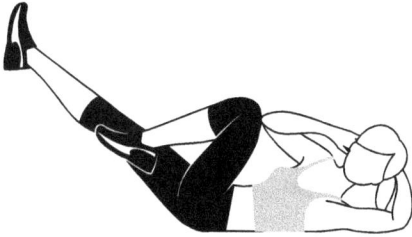

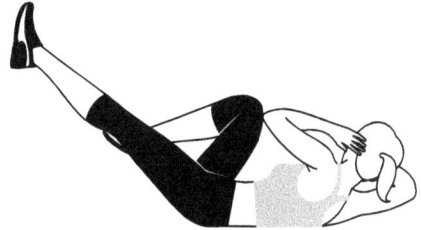

Lie face up and place your hands behind your head, supporting your neck with your fingers. Make sure your core is tight and the small of your back is pushed hard against the floor. Lift your knees in toward your chest while lifting your shoulder blades off the floor. Rotate to the right, bringing the left elbow towards the right knee as you extend the other leg into the air. Switch sides, bringing the right elbow towards the left knee. Alternate each side in a pedalling motion.

Leg RAISE

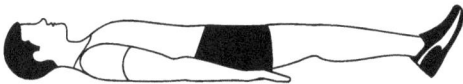

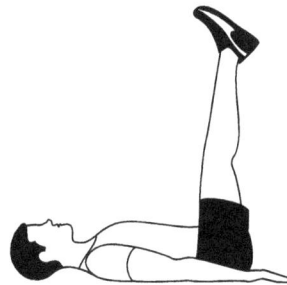

Lie on your back. Place your hands, palms down, on the floor beside you. Raise your legs off the ground (exhale as you go) until your toes are pointing to the ceiling and your legs are straight. Keep your knees locked throughout the exercise. Hold for 2 secs then lower your legs to approximately 6 inches from the floor before raising then again.

Standing SIDE CRUNCH

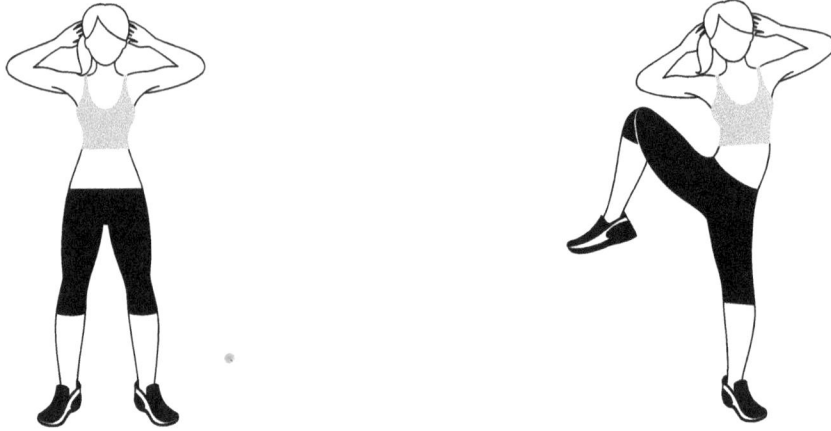

Stand with feet shoulder-width apart, core engaged and knees slightly bent. Lift your right leg, bending the knee 90 degrees and turning thigh out to side. Place both hands behind your head and crunch your right elbow to your right knee. Alternate between legs.

T-STABILISATION

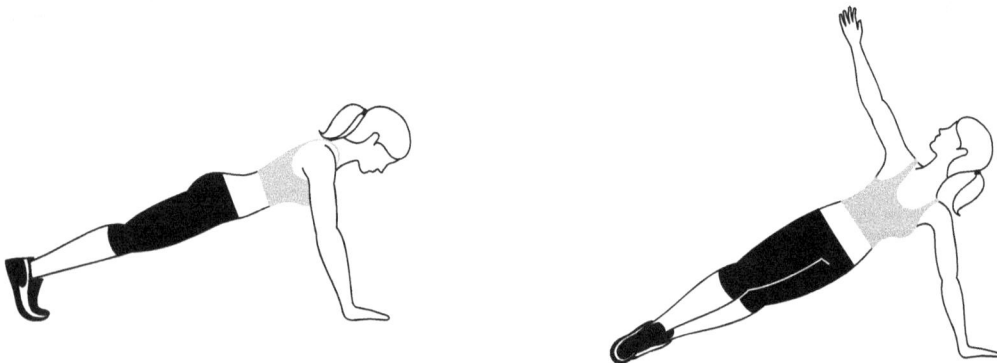

Assume a standard push-up position. Lift your right arm up as you rotate your body to the right using your right leg to cross your left for balance. Rotate all the way over until your arm is straight up and your left side is facing the ground. Your body will now look like a "T" on its side. Hold this position for 5 secs. Reverse movements back to starting position. Repeat on opposite side.

Jumping JACKS

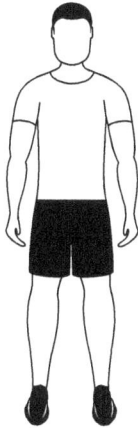

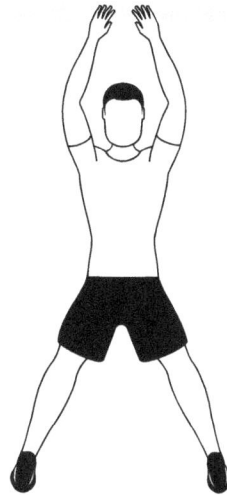

Stand with your feet together and your hands down by your side. In one motion jump your feet out to the side and raise your arms above your head. Immediately reverse by jumping back to the starting position.

V-UP

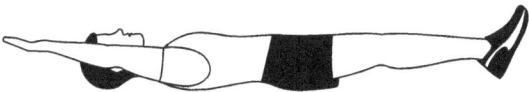

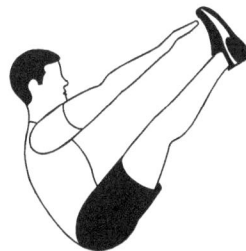

Lay flat on the floor with your legs straight and your arms extended over your head. Lift your chest and legs up off the ground in unison. Your chest should be led by your arms. You should aim to touch your toes at the top of each repetition. As you touch your toes, the top of your tail bone should be the only thing in contact with the ground.

Core WORKOUT TWO

- Exercise 1: **SIT UP** 30 secs | 10 secs rest
- Exercise 2: **FLUTTER KICK** 30 secs | 10 secs rest
- Exercise 3: **WINDSHIELD WIPERS** 30 secs | 10 secs rest
- Exercise 4: **MOUNTAIN CLIMBER** 30 secs | 10 secs rest
- Exercise 5: **SUPERMAN** 30 secs | 10 secs rest
- Exercise 6: **PLANK JACK** 30 secs | 2 minute rest

Repeat for 2 more sets

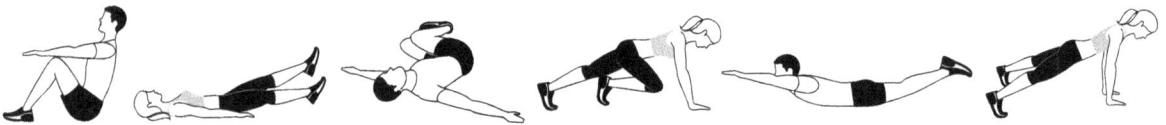

Perform each exercise as many times as possible within 30 seconds or hold for the desired length of time depending on the drill. Rest for 10 seconds then perform the next exercise again for 30 secs with a 10 sec rest in between exercises. Repeat until all 6 exercises have been completed.

Rest for 2 minutes then repeat the whole set two more times with a 2 minute rest in between.

Sit UP

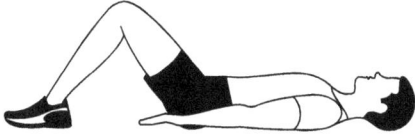

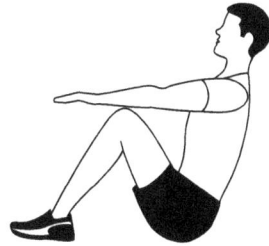

Lie on your back with your knees bent and your arms extended at your sides. and your feet flat on the floor. Engage your core and slowly curl your upper back off the floor towards your knees with your arms extended out. Roll back down to the starting position.

Flutter KICK

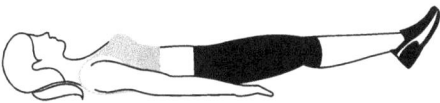

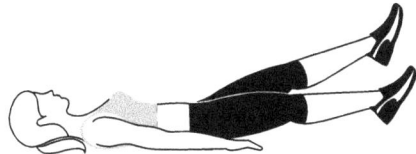

Lie on your back with legs straight and extend your arms by your sides. Lift your heels about 6 inches and quickly kick your feet up and down in a scissor-like motion.

Windshield WIPERS

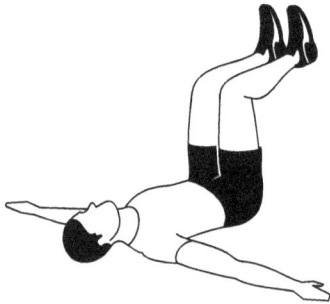

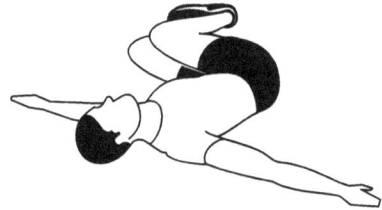

Lie on your back with your arms straight out to the sides. Lift your legs and bend the knees at a 90-degree angle. Rotate the hips to one side without letting the legs touch the floor. Lift your legs and return to the starting position. Rotate the hips to the opposite side and repeat.

Mountain CLIMBER

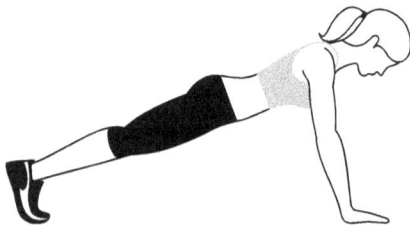

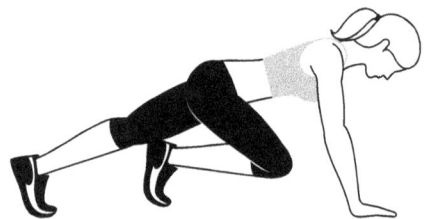

Begin in a pushup position, with your weight supported by your hands and toes. Flexing the knee and hip, bring one leg towards the corresponding arm. Explosively reverse the positions of your legs, extending the bent leg until the leg is straight and supported by the toe, and bringing the other foot up with the hip and knee flexed. Repeat in an alternating fashion.

Superman

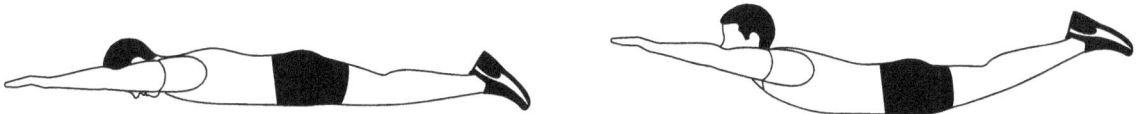

Lie straight and face down on the floor. Simultaneously raise your arms, legs, and chest off of the floor and hold this position for 2 seconds. Slowly begin to lower your arms, legs and chest back down to the starting position while inhaling.

Plank JACK

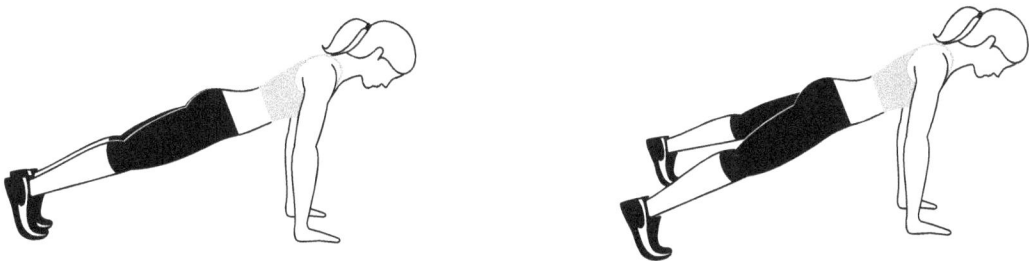

Start in the plank position with more weight resting on your forearms. The body should form a straight line from the shoulders to the ankles. Engage your core then jump the feet out to the sides as if you were performing a jumping jack but keep the upper body still. Return to the starting position and repeat.

Core WORKOUT THREE

- Exercise 1: **PULSE UPS** 30 secs | 10 secs rest
- Exercise 2: **REVERSE PLANK** 30 secs | 10 secs rest
- Exercise 3: **HIGH KNEES** 30 secs | 10 secs rest
- Exercise 4: **RUSSIAN TWIST** 30 secs | 10 secs rest
- Exercise 5: **L SIT** Hold position for as long as possible | start with 2 sec holds | 10 secs rest
- Exercise 6: **SIDE PLANK LEG LIFT** 15 secs on each side | 2 minute rest

• Repeat for 2 more sets

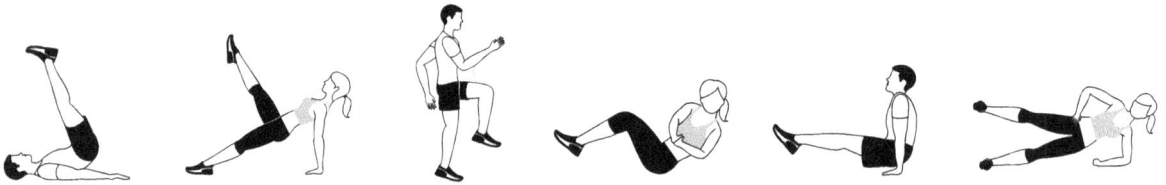

Perform each exercise as many times as possible within 30 seconds or hold for the desired length of time depending on the drill. Rest for 10 seconds then perform the next exercise again for 30 secs with a 10 sec rest in between exercises. Repeat until all 6 exercises have been completed.

Rest for 2 minutes then repeat the whole set two more times with a 2 minute rest in between.

Pulse UPS

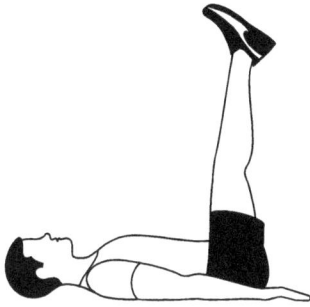

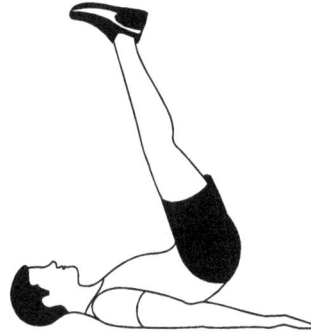

Lie flat on the ground and place your hands at your sides. Raise your legs vertically upwards so that that they are perpendicular to the floor. Start raising your upper body by contracting your core and reaching out for the legs. Feel a squeeze in your abdominal muscles and glutes. Return to the starting position.

Reverse PLANK

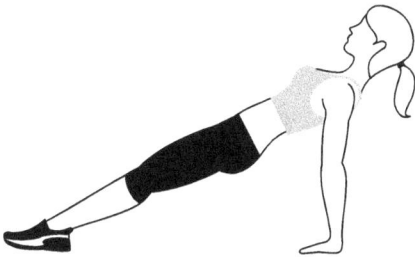

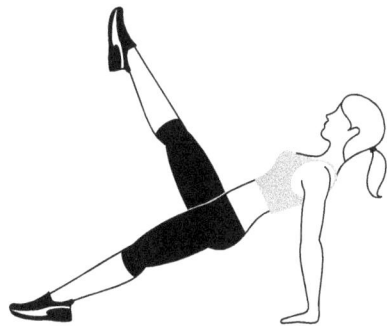

Sit tall with both your legs extended. Place your hands flat to the floor behind you, fingers facing in. Press into your hands and feet to raise your torso, forming a straight line from your head to your toes. Lift your right leg to the ceiling and hold for 3 secs. Return your right leg to the floor then lift the leg again holding for 3 secs in raised position.

High KNEES

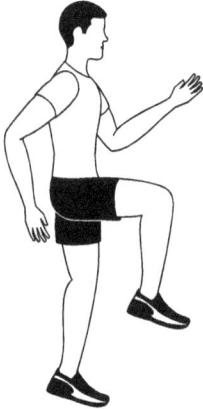

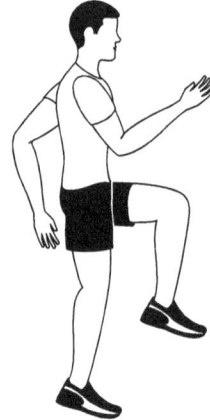

Stand straight with the feet hip width apart, looking straight ahead and arms hanging down by your side. Jump from one foot to the other at the same time lifting your knees as high as possible, hip height is advisable. The arms should be following the motion. Try holding your hands just above the hips so that your knees touch the palms of your hands as you lift your knees.

Russian TWIST

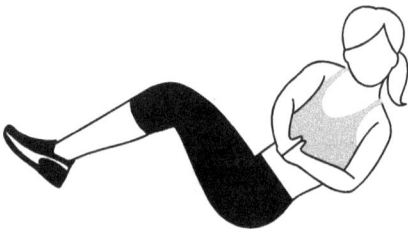

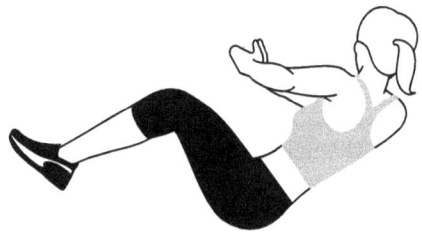

Sit on the floor with your hips and knees bent 90 degrees with arms extended and hands clasped and your back straight (your torso should be at about 45 degrees to the floor). Explosively twist your torso as far as you can to the left and then reverse the motion, twisting as far as you can to the right.

L-SIT

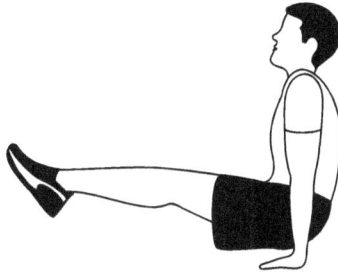

Sit on the floor with your hands directly under your shoulders, fingers facing forward. From this position, push into the floor with your hands, straighten your arms, and bring your shoulders down in order to lift your tail bone off the floor. Hold this position. Begin by holding for just a few seconds then as you grow stronger, progress to longer periods aiming for 15-30 second holds.

Side Plank LEG LIFT

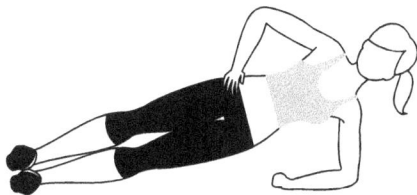

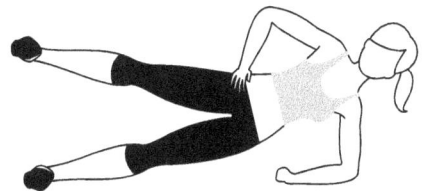

Place your left elbow on the ground. Keeping your spine lengthened and your abs engaged, lift your right leg up just higher than your top hip. Keep your waist up and lifted, and don't let your upper body drop in to your bottom shoulder. Return your leg to the starting position. Repeat for 15 seconds then change position so your right elbow is on the ground lifting your left leg.

Cobra STRETCH

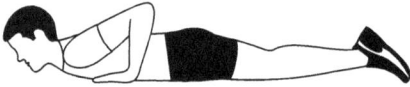

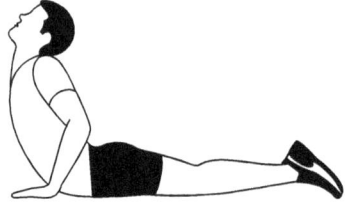

Lay on your stomach with your palms facing down and positioned right underneath your shoulders. Keep your legs shoulder-width apart. Pushing down with your hands, lift your chest as you exhale. Be sure to keep your hips and the tops of your feet firmly planted on the floor. You should feel a rewarding stretch in your core. Slowly lower your chest back to floor. Repeat 5 times.

Cat Cow STRETCH

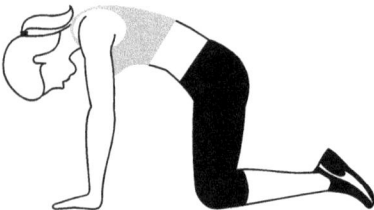

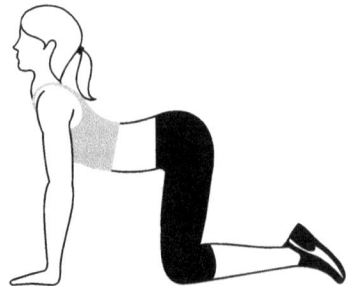

Begin with your hands and knees on the floor. Exhale while rounding your spine up towards the ceiling, pulling your belly button up towards your spine, and engaging your core. Inhale while arching your back and letting your tummy relax. Repeat 5 times.

www.ingramcontent.com/pod-product-compliance
Lightning Source LLC
Chambersburg PA
CBHW081257040426
42452CB00014B/2546